THE PENICILLIN GROUP OF DRUGS

THE PENICILLIN GROUP
OF DRUGS

BY

GORDON T. STEWART

Professor of Epidemiology and Pathology,
University of North Carolina, Chapel Hill, N.C. (U.S.A.)

ELSEVIER PUBLISHING COMPANY
AMSTERDAM – LONDON – NEW YORK
1965

ELSEVIER PUBLISHING COMPANY
335 JAN VAN GALENSTRAAT, P.O. BOX 211, AMSTERDAM

AMERICAN ELSEVIER PUBLISHING COMPANY, INC.
52 VANDERBILT AVENUE, NEW YORK, N.Y. 10017

ELSEVIER PUBLISHING COMPANY LIMITED
RIPPLESIDE COMMERCIAL ESTATE, BARKING, ESSEX

LIBRARY OF CONGRESS CATALOG CARD NUMBER 65-13899

WITH 11 ILLUSTRATIONS AND 17 TABLES

PRINTED IN THE NETHERLANDS

To My Family

PREFACE

This book was begun in England and completed in America. It is, therefore, my pleasure to acknowledge the help and encouragement which I have received from colleagues on both sides of the Atlantic. In England, my interest in penicillin dates from 1944 when, as one of the first (and most ignorant) "Penicillin officers" in the Royal Navy, I was initiated into problems of production, assay and usage at the R. N. Medical School, Clevedon, by Surgeon Commander C. A. Green, R.N.V.R., now Professor of Bacteriology at the University of Durham. Subsequently, I had the privilege while working at the Wright–Fleming Institute of Microbiology in London of contact with Sir Alexander Fleming who did not often talk about penicillin but laid more emphasis than anyone I have known upon personal experimentation and observation. He was a man whose extreme reticence concealed a great depth of kindliness, sincerity and sagacity but few of the younger people seemed to appreciate this. Among those few, I must mention Dr. Amelia Voureka (Lady Fleming), herself an able bacteriologist, whose understanding of her husband's qualities contributed largely to the biography written so ably by M. André Maurois. For information about earlier events, I have to thank Professors R. Hare, W. D. Newcomb, M. Pryce and Dr. W. H. Hughes.

The contribution of the Sir William Dunn School of Pathology at Oxford to the development of penicillins and cephalosporins is incalculable. I hope that, in these pages, I have indicated the significance of the continuing interest of this School in fundamental aspects of antibiotic activity. I am personally indebted to Professor Ernst Chain for his interest, as well as to other present and past members of the Dunn School, notably Professor E. P. Abraham, Dr. N. G. Heatley and Dr. G. G. F. Newton for helpful discussions of past events and present trends, as well as for samples of cephalosporins when supplies were scarce.

The greater part of the book is concerned with the newer penicillins which arose out of a programme planned by Chain and the Beecham Research

Laboratories Ltd. Having enjoyed for six years close collaboration with the Beecham research team, I find it difficult to confine my thanks to a few individuals but in thanking the late Dr. John Farquharson, Mr. F. P. Doyle, Mr. F. R. Batchelor, Dr. E. T. Knudsen, Dr. J. H. C. Nayler and Dr. G. N. Rolinson, I am trying to thank the whole management and staff and, at the same time, paying tribute to the immense benefits arising from this kind of research by the pharmaceutical industry. It is especially pleasing to note the recent recognition of Beecham's achievement by the award of the Gold Medal of the Most Sacred Society of Apothecaries to Mr. Doyle and Dr. Rolinson. Among other organisations, I must thank the National Research Development Corporation and Glaxo Research Ltd. for supplying me with cephalosporins and the Connaught Research Laboratories, Messrs. Pfizer, Boots and others for supplying me with various derivatives of 6-APA.

My own recent work in the antibiotic field has been carried out mainly at Carshalton and I am glad of this opportunity to register my gratitude to many colleagues there, in Queen Mary's Hospital for Children and in the Medical Research Council's Laboratories. Again it is difficult to confine my thanks to a few names, but I owe special acknowledgement firstly to my chief assistant Mr. R. J. Holt, whose technical collaboration has been invaluable; also to Dr. J. M. Barnes, Dr. H. M. T. Coles, Dr. S. Duckett, Miss Patricia Harrison, Dr. R. L. Newman and Mr. H. H. Nixon; and my secretary there, Mrs. Eileen Hardy. I am indebted also to Dr. M. T. Parker, Dr. Patricia Jevons and Professor R. E. O. Williams for their collaborative work with staphylococci extending over several years in the Central Public Health Laboratories at Colindale.

In America, I have encountered many colleagues who have stimulated my interest in less familiar aspects of antibiotic research. In the first place, I must thank the National Science Foundation for bringing me here as a Visiting Foreign Scientist. Numerous new colleagues have opened doorways for me at the University of North Carolina to widen my interest in the control of infection. The Squibb and Bristol pharmaceutical companies, among others, have furnished information about past and present research on penicillins. I have also met some of the pioneers of antibiotic research in America, all of whom have provided useful information, often unique. The manuscript for the later chapters was typed by Mrs. Natalie Harbin and Mrs. Carolyn Owen who assisted also in revision, along with my daughter Linda.

Elsewhere in the world, I find myself indebted also. Dr. W. R. Lane of the Commonwealth Serum Laboratories in Australia generously exchanged information with me about the toxicity to tissue cultures of some of the newer penicillins. Colleagues in Canada, Denmark, Germany, Norway and Poland have sent me strains of bacteria with unusual forms of penicillin resistance which have extended my experience of this problem.

In writing this book, I have become increasingly aware of the beautiful—if accidental—continuity of research and achievement in the subject. The point has now been reached where the benefits to preventive and therapeutic medicine stemming from the β-lactam antibiotics are matched by a scientific understanding which cannot fail to contribute immensely to genetics, pharmacology, microbiology and epidemiology. My own comprehension of these subjects is limited, but I have enjoyed pulling some of the strings together for I find that science is more satisfying when I glimpse its unity. The story of these antibiotics illustrates a continuing interaction of intellectual and practical endeavour, and this is what the book is about.

Lake Shore Drive,   GORDON T. STEWART
Chapel Hill, N.C.
June 1965

G.T. STEWART, *The Penicillin Group of Drugs*

Elsevier Publishing Company, Amsterdam, 1965

ERRATUM

p. 203, first column:

7-Aminopenicillanic acid, *see* 7-ACA

should read:

7-Aminocephalosporanic acid, *see* 7-ACA

CONTENTS

Chapter 1

DISCOVERY IN 1929

*Discovery is seeing what everybody has seen,
and thinking what nobody has thought.*

CLAUDE BERNARD

Great thoughts and great deeds can occur at any time and any place, but great discoveries are dependent on people and places. Paddington is a bustling, nondescript place in West London, best known for its railway terminus and, to a much lesser extent, for the hospital standing almost next door. But it was in this hospital, at the turn of the century, that an Irishman in his early forties named Almroth Wright, who had been educated in Europe, established a small department of research which was to become one of the first nurseries for the infant science of bacteriology in England. The seed of discovery was planted in this nursery by Wright, best remembered as a forceful eccentric who believed that something could and should be done about communicable disease.

The hospital, St. Mary's, was and is unlike the traditional teaching hospitals of London. Many of its students were of middle class origin, often from Wales; the staff were, likewise, heterogeneous, and newcomers were usually welcomed. In this setting, Wright was able to create something much greater than a department of inoculation and research, unusual as that was at the time: he formed a school of thought. It was this school which fostered the philosophy originated by Metchnikoff of direct observation of the mechanism of natural defence against infection, and of the practicability of prevention and cure. It was to this school that several thoughtful men were attracted in their formative years, among them Alexander Fleming, who was a naturalist as well as a doctor. It was in this school that his mind was prepared for the observation that led to the discovery of penicillin.

The characters of Wright and those who worked and argued with him in London were essential elements in the discovery and preliminary examination of penicillin. Like all great men, Wright had many strings in his bow. From his own writings[1], from contemporary literature, and from subsequent character studies by Colebrook[2], Maurois[3] and Hare[4], as well as from the vivid recollections of those who knew him, there emerges a vigorous and varied personality who could display humour and gentleness along with

References p. 7

ferocity and impatience; he worked hard himself, at the bench and in his consulting room, for he believed that doctors in laboratories should also see patients, and encouraged his assistants to do so. His intellectual interests and gifts were wide—from poetry to bacteriology—but his outlook was largely pragmatic and his research was applied with constancy to the prevention and cure of infection by methods utilising natural substances. His belief, to which he clung obstinately, was that prevention of infection could be achieved by immunisation and cure by stimulating the various components of the body's natural defences, or by administering these components; his own achievements—demonstrating the natural bactericidal power of the blood and the presence of opsonins—together with his own eloquence and determination, convinced many of his associates that his approach was rational and likely to be fruitful. Events to date have proved him wrong; pioneer as he was in immunology, Wright did not himself discover any therapeutic substance of lasting value.

Nevertheless, today, the Research Department at St. Mary's is renamed the "Wright–Fleming Institute of Microbiology" in recognition of these two key figures in a long chapter which culminated and ended with the early description of penicillin. Wright's importance—in this discovery and in the broader subject of microbiology—was as the founder of a productive and provocative school of thought; he saw the ravages of communicable disease as a challenge to his humanity as well as to his scientific curiosity; and he imbued others, inside and outside his department, with the credulity of his belief. It is no discredit to the other members of the research department, several of whom became distinguished by their own efforts and a few of whom are alive today, to say that no one there except Wright could have given such impetus to these particular researches.

A book on penicillins would be incomplete without recounting this background. Research is now a commonplace, almost a routine, but discovery is still a rarity which can only be understood fully in terms of people and places. It is often said that research workers need isolation and tranquillity; this may be true of some subjects, but the school which unearthed the leading clue to antibiotic therapy was crowded, controversial and as much a part of the motley borough of Paddington as the stale air which yielded the penicillium mould, not inappropriately, on a plate.

Alexander Fleming was born in 1881, the seventh son of a working farmer, at Lochfield, Ayrshire, Scotland. He attended first the village elementary school at Lochfield, then a larger school at Darvel, to which he journeyed on foot, four miles each way each day. At the age of twelve he was sent to

Kilmarnock Academy, returning home at week-ends. When he was fourteen, like many other Scottish country boys, he left school and went to London, joining three of his brothers there, to earn his living. One of his brothers, Tom, who had studied medicine at Glasgow University, was now in practice in London, and found room for Alec, two other brothers and a sister, in his house.

After a brief spell of study at the Polytechnic School, Alec took a post as junior clerk in a shipping company, the American Line, in Leadenhall Street. When the Boer War broke out in 1900, he joined the London Scottish Regiment as a private, along with two of his brothers. At the age of twenty he inherited a legacy of £250 from an uncle and, with encouragement from his doctor brother, Tom, decided to study medicine. He sat the entrance examination of the College of Preceptors and, in 1901, entered St. Mary's Hospital Medical School. As a student he had a distinguished record; when qualified, he prepared for a surgical career by acquiring the Fellowship of the Royal College of Surgeons. He was, however, persuaded by Dr. John Freeman to apply for a post in the Inoculation Department. Wright in 1908 accepted him as a trainee in bacteriology and there he was to remain for the rest of his life. Shortly before this, he had declared his interest in communicable disease by writing an essay on "Acute bacterial infections" which won him the Cheadle gold medal offered by the School.

For the next four years, Fleming studied and applied Wright's immunological techniques but, unlike Wright, he accepted chemotherapy rather than immunotherapy as a means of treating infection. He was one of the first men in England to use Ehrlich's newly-discovered arsphenamine ("salvarsan") in the treatment of syphilis[5], possibly because his hands were safer than those of his colleagues in delivering this highly-irritant drug intravenously. In 1914 he became a medical officer in the Royal Army Medical Corps and served, under Wright, in a laboratory at Boulogne-sur-Mer, established for the purpose of devising methods to control wound infection. His practical experience of this appalling problem, and his interest, deepened beyond words. He drew attention to the role of necrotic tissue in facilitating wound infection[6] and devised methods for the rational use of irrigation, antiseptics and transfusion; he was particularly impressed by the failure of all available antiseptics to sterilise wounds without damaging tissue or killing leucocytes[7].

After the war Fleming, now married, returned to the Research Department at St. Mary's Hospital. In 1922 he described the bacteriolytic substance[8] (christened "lysozyme" by Wright) in mucus, tears and other secretions as well as in egg albumin, plants and skin. With Allison and Ridley he attempted to extract and purify the active principle but without success[9], though he maintained his interest in lysozyme and said in later years that it could be "more important than penicillin". He showed also that lysozyme was present in phagocytes and that staphylococci could acquire resistance to it on exposure[10].

The story of Fleming's chance observation that a contaminant mould of the *Penicillium* family produced a substance inhibitory to staphylococci is now a classic. His frame of mind at the time and his subsequent activities are less well recognised, though no less important than the chance observation. Maurois[3] gives an excellent description of what happened, based on the recollections of eye-witnesses. It is clear that, in Fleming's well-prepared mind, the importance of the observation was soon registered: not only did he take the essential steps of testing and preserving the mould; he also gave up many other activities so that he could concentrate his attention on the phenomenon which he had encountered. It is fortunate for mankind that he had the intelligence and the opportunity to do so, though he has been criticised—by those who knew and loved him best, as well as by others—for not mustering more energy in his research. He knew that chemical knowledge was the answer to his problem; but he never attempted to learn any more chemistry himself, leaving this part of the problem uncritically to others.

This was in 1928, and the phenomenon known as antibiosis had already been described by many scientists, including Lister[11] (1871), Roberts[12] (1874), Tyndall[13] (1876), Pasteur and Joubert[14] (1877) and several others. *Penicillium* had in fact already been used by Gossio[15] in 1896 to produce an antibacterial substance. The therapeutic possibilities of antibiosis—the word seems first to have been used in France—appealed to French scientists, who have always been attracted by medicinal substances of natural origin. At the end of the 19th century, research was proceeding on those lines, but nothing useful was produced. An occurrence such as that which Fleming witnessed must have been observed and even deliberately produced many times; the importance lay less in Fleming's observation than in his action. Being at heart a good Presbyterian, he felt in an entirely unpretentious way that Destiny entered his laboratory that day; not least among his endearing qualities was his candid admission, years later, that "the fates were wonderfully kind to me"[16].

Fleming then proceeded to test other fungi, including eight strains of *Penicillium*, for antibiotic production. The only species which produced a bactericidal substance was a strain of *Penicillium* identical in appearance and properties to the original mould which was identified at that time as *P. rubrum*, though in subsequent studies it was reclassified by Thom as *P. notatum*. He characterised the antibiotic, accurately, as being soluble in water and ethanol, insoluble in chloroform and ether, stable at pH 6.8, and moderately stable to heat. In his first paper on the subject[17] published in the following year in the *British Journal of Experimental Pathology*, he described in detail the rate and extent of bactericidal activity and noted that the action of penicillin was directed essentially against gram-positive and gram-negative pyogenic cocci, there being little or no action on gram-negative bacilli. For this reason, he was impressed by the immediate practicability of incorporating penicillin to make blood agar selective for the isolation of *Haemophilus* in sputum. This was featured in the title of his paper "On the antibacterial action of cultures of a penicillium, with special reference to their use in the isolation of B. influenzae". The title might have been chosen better, for it gave rise to the impression, then and later, that Fleming was not aware of the therapeutic potential of his discovery. The text of the paper belies this, for he mentions the lack of toxicity of the antibacterial substance, which he named penicillin, in the rabbit, mouse, human eye, human leucocytes and wound surfaces. It is also clear, in the paper and in notes made soon after, that he tested the therapeutic properties of the crude brew of penicillin in wounds infected with staphylococci. Attempts to purify it by evaporation *in vacuo*, performed by his colleagues Stuart Craddock and Frederick Ridley, were unsuccessful. A report presented to the Medical Research Club evoked no questions or interest from anyone in the audience.

Fleming then approached other chemists, including Harold King, head of the department of chemistry at the Medical Research Council's Laboratories at Hampstead. Independently, the Professor of Biochemistry at the London School of Hygiene and Tropical Medicine, Harold Raistrick, studied penicillin with the help of a bacteriologist, R. Lovell, and another chemist, P. W. Clutterbuck. They succeeded in isolating the inert pigment from the mould, but not the antibacterial substance. Their work[18] came to a halt with Clutterbuck's untimely death.

Meanwhile Fleming had published another paper dealing with the use of penicillin as a selective agent in media for the isolation of *Haemophilus*[19]. In 1932, when it was clear that attempts at chemical extraction and purification were fruitless, he published an account of his use of the crude brew as a topical agent in the treatment of infected wounds[20]. He gave a paper and a demonstration about penicillin to the 2nd International Congress of Microbiology[21] in 1936, and continued to speak to other scientists about the

References p. 7

importance of purifying it by chemical means, but again failed to arouse any obvious interest.

To anyone interested in the evolution of medical science, these happenings in 1929–32 are most revealing. Many medical men saw no possibility—or refused to see any possibility—of treating any major bacterial infection by a drug, though the practicability of systemic chemotherapy had already been demonstrated in syphilis and, with empirical remedies, in malaria and amoebic dysentery. And yet, in every general hospital, and especially in children's wards, bacterial infection was by far the greatest challenge to the therapeutic impotence of the day. Since the days of Lister, antiseptics had come and gone. None was fit to swallow or inject, though Browning, following Ehrlich's approach, had found the flavine acridines to be less toxic than most antiseptics. Hindsight is an easy road to wisdom, but it is nevertheless astonishing to reflect that no one at the time, except Raistrick and an American bacteriologist, R. D. Reid[22] of Baltimore, exhibited active interest in any of Fleming's reports, though to any bacteriologist in those days an impure but non-toxic filtrate killing staphylococci at a dilution of 1 : 600 must have offered the prospect of a strange new experience. Academic research in medicine is often too fundamental to be concerned with the prevention and cure of disease but, even in sympathetic circles, Fleming's work aroused no interest, nor was there any evidence of exploratory action on the part of the pharmaceutical industry. There are fashions in medical science no less than in costumes; Fleming's observations, reported at a time when therapeutic nihilism was the vogue, were completely ignored. Even Wright, to whom research on infection was a religion, was oblivious to the therapeutic potential of Fleming's work, though perhaps appreciative of its technical accuracy.

Some personal factors also have to be considered. Though shrewd in his assessment of men and matters, Fleming was abrupt in manner and devoid of guile; he was also habitually taciturn and an indifferent speaker. Within himself he was wise and surprisingly far-seeing, but in address he seldom pressed a point and was not persuasive. At St. Mary's he had long been respected, even popular, for his sincerity, even temper and athletic ability, but he failed to convince anyone there that research on penicillin should be effectively supported or even repeated. The despotism of Wright may have been an adverse factor here, for Fleming often acknowledged the co-operation of some of his clinical colleagues who allowed him to treat their patients[22]. But this co-operation almost certainly was given to Fleming the doctor rather than to penicillin the drug. Nevertheless, some useful cases came his way[23, 24] and a controlled trial at that time might have disclosed more objectively the therapeutic activity of penicillin; even in the crude brew applied topically, there was enough antibacterial potency to eliminate sensitive organisms from burns, wounds, ocular and other localised infections; but Fleming, like Wright, was distrustful of trends and statistics. Seeing was believing; had they thought otherwise, penicillin might never have been seen.

It must be remembered that biochemistry, wherein lay the solution of Fleming's technical difficulties, was a younger science even than bacteriology. Techniques which are familiar now to undergraduate students were then undeveloped. In these circumstances, wittingly or unwittingly, Fleming probably did the best thing he could do in describing, simply and factually, his basic findings; he set the stage admirably for a subsequent performance by a more expert team who read the literature wisely.

REFERENCES

[1] WRIGHT, A. E., *Prolegomena to the logic which searches for Truth*, Heinemann, London, 1941.
[2] COLEBROOK, L., *Almroth Wright*, Heinemann, London, 1954.
[3] MAUROIS, A., *The Life of Sir Alexander Fleming*, Jonathan Cape, London, 1959.
[4] HARE, R., *Almroth Edward Wright*, A centenary lecture given at the Wright–Fleming Institute, Oct. 31, 1961.
[5] FLEMING, A. AND COLEBROOK, L., *Lancet, i* (1911) 1631.
[6] FLEMING, A., *Lancet, ii* (1915) 538.
[7] WRIGHT, A. E., FLEMING, A. AND COLEBROOK, L., *Lancet, i* (1918) 831.
[8] WRIGHT, A. E., *Proc. roy. Soc. B.*, *93* (1922) 306.
[9] WRIGHT, A. E. AND ALLISON, V. D., *Brit. J. exp. Path.*, *3* (1922) 252.
[10] WRIGHT, A. E. AND ALLISON, V. D., *Brit. J. exp. Path.*, *8* (1927) 214.
[11] LISTER, J., *Commonplace Book*, 1871, entry of Nov. 25; recorded in *Ann. roy. Coll. Surg. Engl.*, *6* (1950).
[12] ROBERTS, W., *Phil. Trans. B.*, *164* (1874) 457.
[13] TYNDALL, J., *Phil. Trans. B.*, *166* (1876) 27.
[14] PASTEUR, L. AND JOUBERT, J. E., *C.R. Acad. Sci. (Paris)*, *85* (1877) 101.
[15] GOSSIO, B., *Riv. Iq. San. pub.*, *7* (1896) 825, 961.
[16] FLEMING, A., *Harv. Publ. Hlth. Alumni Bull.*, *47* (1945) 580.
[17] FLEMING, A., *Brit. J. exp. Path.*, *10* (1929) 226.
[18] CLUTTERBUCK, P. W., LOVELL, R. AND RAISTRICK, H., *Biochem. J.*, *26* (1932) 1907.
[19] FLEMING, A. AND MACLEAN, I. H., *Brit. J. exp. Path.*, *11* (1930) 127.
[20] FLEMING, A., *J. Path. Bact.*, *35* (1932) 831.
[21] FLEMING, A., *Proceedings of the second International Congress of Microbiology*, (1937) p. 33.
[22] REID, R. D., *J. Bact.*, *29* (1935) 215.
[23] FLEMING, A., *The Medical Society's Transactions*, London, *64* (1945) 142.
[24] WRIGHT, A. D., *The Medical Society's Transactions*, London, *64* (1945) 145.

Chapter 2

TEN YEARS LATER: 1939 AND AFTER

The clever men at Oxford
Know all there is to be knowed.

SONG (K. GRAHAME)

If the first key figure in the discovery of penicillin was a scientific naturalist, the second was a natural scientist, a pathologist with the outlook of a physiologist. Howard Florey, who was born and educated in Australia, became interested in natural antibacterial mechanisms while working in the University Department of Pathology at Sheffield in the early thirties[1]. He confirmed and extended Fleming's work on lysozyme and, when he moved to the Chair of Pathology at Oxford, planned a programme of research on natural antibacterial substances. Among those who joined his staff in Oxford was Ernst Chain, born in Berlin in 1906. With other members of Florey's department, Chain continued the study of lysozyme which was purified and crystallised[2,3] by 1938. Various other antibacterial substances were also investigated, including pyocyanase (whose bactericidal properties had first been described by Emmerich in 1902), actinomycetin and penicillin. It was obvious from Fleming's original paper that penicillin was one of the most promising antibacterial agents ever described among about forty references read in a preliminary survey of the literature. Chain believed that its instability, which had baffled Raistrick[4], was not an insuperable difficulty. Fleming's experiments were quickly repeated and confirmed, and preparations made for growing the mould on a larger scale to fathom the biochemical depth of this marker of bacterial antagonism.

Meanwhile, the climate of opinion had become more favourable toward chemotherapy. Domagk's description of the bacteriostatic properties of prontosil[5] in the Bayer laboratories in Germany, and the subsequent isolation of the active principle *p*-aminobenzene sulphonamide by workers at the Pasteur Institut in Paris[6] established the fact that pyogenic bacteria could be suppressed *in vivo*, while clinical studies conducted in France, Germany, England, and elsewhere by various workers[5-8], demonstrated in a few months that complete cure of severe streptococcal infections was practicable. Within a year the efficacy of sulphonamide in gonorrhoea, bacterial pneumonia, meningitis and other conditions caused a revolution which altered therapeutic outlook no less than procedure, while the synthesis of new derivatives proved that pharmacological drawbacks in the primary sulphonamide could be overcome. To anyone studying medicine at that time, the somersault in therapeutic thinking was quite spectacular. In research circles, however, this channelled thinking in the direction of synthesis, not antibiosis. In selecting their subject, the Oxford workers followed the new fashion but, in their approach to it, they swam against the tide, as they were soon to find.

In their early work on the cultivation of *P. notatum* in 1939, the Oxford workers used simple Czapek–Dox medium, still a favourite for this purpose. They accelerated growth by adding a boiled extract of yeast and they increased the yield of penicillin by harvesting and replacing the medium beneath the surface mat of fungus, though this procedure was eventually abandoned because of the liability to contamination. To extract the penicillin, they used a solvent-transfer process based on the technique of Clutterbuck, Lovell and Raistrick and produced early in 1940 small quantities of a brown powder which inhibited the growth of *Staphylococcus aureus* at dilutions of 1 in 2 million. This powder probably contained less than 2% of penicillin but, even so, it was remarkably non-toxic in animals. When John Barnes, now a well-known toxicologist, gave the first intravenous injection to a mouse, he remarked to Chain that the new substance was at least non-toxic, if less colourful, than pyocyanin, which was still an object of departmental interest; but further toxicology and protection tests in mice infected with β-haemolytic streptococci left no one in any doubt over the therapeutic potential of the crude penicillin which thereafter became the dominant subject of study[9].

The next problem was large-scale production and extraction. The descriptions of Heatley[10] and others[11,12] hint at some of the difficulties experienced in overcoming this problem in a small University department in war-time, but modestly understate the ingenuity and determination of the team which amassed culture vessels, bedpans, ceramic slipware and other utensils for the purpose, and devised a counter-current solvent extraction which yielded, early in 1941, enough penicillin for a preliminary study in human subjects. The cup-plate assay technique developed by Heatley led to the definition of the Oxford unit of activity (0.6 μg of pure penicillin G), still in use today.

The first clinical trial with the crude penicillin powder was conducted on 12th February, 1941. The patient was an Oxford policeman, dying of staphylococcal osteomyelitis and pyaemia in the Radcliffe Infirmary, Oxford. Penicillin arrested the infection almost immediately and the patient showed signs of recovery; but, 5 days later, when all the penicillin had been used, the infection resumed its advance and killed the patient. There are times in human affairs when tragedy clears the path, and this fatality, providing two trials in a sense for the price of one, emphasised the need and the urgency for further research upon production. Enough penicillin was produced at Oxford during the next few weeks for the treatment of five other patients, four of them children, with staphylococcal or streptococcal infections which had not responded to sulphonamides or surgical measures. The results[13] were convincing, each in a different way, and the absence of toxicity was almost as impressive as the rapid therapeutic effect. In the present day, when a clinical trial is becoming an exercise in statistics and bureaucracy, there is irony in the reflection that the massive efforts which followed were based upon a few toxicity tests in rodents (Fig. 1) and upon a clinical trial in six selected subjects, two of whom died. Had the toxicity tests been extended to guinea pigs, penicillin might have been rejected; had current regulations been in force, it would have been ineligible for submission.

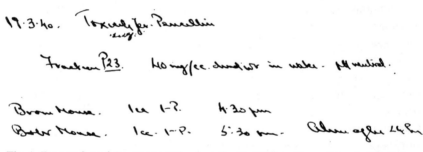

Fig. 1. Excerpt from laboratory notebook at the Sir William Dunn School of Pathology Oxford. (By courtesy of Dr. J. M. Barnes).

The publication in the *Lancet* of the two reports upon penicillin excited more interest than Fleming's paper in 1929, but not much more. At Oxford, Professor Trueta was credited with the remark that, when he saw Florey looking at patients, he knew something unusual was happening; in the burns units at Oxford and Glasgow, penicillin was applied topically in minute quantities to eradicate pyogenic cocci—only to open the road to *Pseudomonas pyocyanea*. Fleming visited Oxford and thereafter obtained some of the brown powder for microbiological and clinical purposes at St. Mary's Hospital. Pleased as he undoubtedly was at the purification of his active principle, he shared the view of many when he stated that penicillin would be almost useless as a therapeutic agent until synthesised[14]. This was the view held also by those in industry who had been approached in 1940. The penicillin content of the crude brew was at most 2 units/ml; 50–80% of this was lost in extraction; hence 2000 litres of fermentation liquor would be required for the treatment of one patient. The future seemed to lie with synthesis but, under the conditions prevailing in Britain during the grim phase of the war in 1940–41, this could not be contemplated, nor could fermentation vats be made available. After consultation with Dr. Weaver of the Rockefeller Foundation it was decided that Florey and Heatley should visit America to see if large-scale production could be contemplated there. With financial support from the Rockefeller Foundation, Florey and Heatley arrived in the United States on July 2nd, 1941.

The phenomenon of antibiosis had not escaped attention in America. Dr. Charles Thom, of the U.S. Department of Agriculture, had classified Fleming's strain of *Penicillium*; several scientists, among them René Dubos and S. A. Waksman, had worked in and around the subject; research workers at Columbia had already interested themselves in, and confirmed[15], the first laboratory report from Oxford. On arrival, Florey and Heatley first explained their problem to a Dr. J. F. Fulton of New Haven. On his advice they then saw Dr. Ross Harrison, chairman of the National Research Council. Next they visited Dr. Charles Thom, the mycologist, at Beltsville, Md., whence they proceeded to the Northern Regional Research Laboratories of the U.S. Department of Agriculture at Peoria, Ill. On July 14th they had detailed discussions there with Dr. O. E. May (Director) and Dr. R. D. Coghill (Fermentation), and it is on record that work on penicillin production began next day, Coghill having suggested that the problem of large-scale production might be answered by deep fermentation. Heatley remained at Peoria for the next six months and research upon production of penicillin soon afterwards became the chief preoccupation of the fermentation division there for the next five years[16,17]. Florey left Peoria after a few days and visited a number of pharmaceutical firms, including Lilly, Connaught, Merck, Sharp & Dohme, Eastman, Squibb, Lederle and Pfizer. Several of these companies showed interest, but the only effective steps towards production at that stage came first from Merck & Co. Inc., then from E. R. Squibb & Sons and Chas. Pfizer & Co. Inc. The ready and incredibly rapid co-operation of these firms, as well as of the U.S. Government, were key factors in the production of penicillin for therapeutic purposes.

August 7th found Florey in Philadelphia talking to A. N. Richards,

References p. 15/16

Professor of Pharmacology at the University of Pennsylvania, with whom he had worked fifteen years previously. Richards had just been appointed chairman of the Committee on Medical Research at the Office of Scientific Research and Development. In Florey's words, Dr. Richards promised to see that "everything possible was done to expedite the production of penicillin", and, under the chairmanship of Dr. Vannevar Bush on October 2nd, the Committee on Medical Research approved this priority. On October 8th a conference was held between representatives of the U.S. Government and four pharmaceutical houses, again under Bush, who was Director of the Office of Scientific Research and Development, as chairman. At this meeting, the firm of Merck agreed to co-operate upon penicillin research and production as a government-sponsored project. The first of many conferences was held on October 20th, with reports from Dr. Thom, Peoria and Merck; it was recommended that the tempo of development be increased further, and the Committee on Medical Research offered, in the first instance, a grant of $8000. At the next conference, on December 17th, it was agreed that all information on research and development from governmental and commercial laboratories should be shared, via the Committee on Medical Research. Much had been achieved since July 2nd when Florey and Heatley arrived in New York; much more was being planned, largely upon the basis of some experimental and clinical results from Oxford. During that same month America entered the war and supplies of penicillin, originally intended for Oxford, were retained in the United States.

At Peoria, where Heatley was still working, Dr. A. J. Moyer had suggested the use of corn-steep liquor which was easier to obtain in bulk than yeast extract. With this and other additions to the culture medium, the yield of penicillin increased from 2 to 40 units/ml, while further improvement was effected by changes of medium, pH conditions and strain of mould. At first Fleming's strain was used, then the Peoria strain NRRL 1249 B2, then (in the course of a widespread search), a strain isolated from a rotten melon bought in the market, NRRL 1951 B25, then an X-ray mutant strain produced at the Carnegie Institute which yielded 500 units/ml, and finally a mutant induced by ultra-violet irradiation at the University of Wisconsin (WIS Q.176) which increased the yield to 900 units/ml. With this diversified approach, and submerged culture, production problems were rapidly being solved. After six months at Peoria, Heatley had moved to the Merck laboratories to place his knowledge at their disposal.

While Florey and Heatley were in America, small-scale production continued at Oxford and two firms (Imperial Chemical Industries Ltd. and then

Kemball, Bishop & Co. Ltd.) began to co-operate. Enough was available in January 1942 to initiate a second clinical trial in which 15 cases were treated by systemic and 172 by local administration of the crude penicillin. The report[18] of this trial should be read in the original, for it shows what can be accomplished under conditions of shortage—of assistance, of money, of apparatus and (not least) of penicillin itself—by critical investigators. The basis of dosage was laid; micro-assay of blood levels, etc. described; oral and parenteral dosage compared; and various clinical factors influencing treatment described. In a child aged 2 months with multiple foci of osteomyelitis "the first good indication of the effective dose . . . was obtained". Twenty years later, this item of clinical history was to be repeated (p. 70). Subsidiary trials of topical therapy were also conducted by Colebrook and others[19] at the Burns Unit in Glasgow Royal Infirmary, by Bodenham[20] at Princess Mary's R.A.F. Hospital, Halton and by Barnes at the Burns Unit in Oxford. The latter two workers used penicillin with sulphanilamide to eradicate pyogenic cocci, a form of therapy which was to prove all-important in the prevention of wound sepsis in battle casualties at later stages in the war. Fleming was impressed by the cure of a case of staphylococcal meningitis treated at St. Mary's Hospital and, with Raistrick, visited the Ministry of Supply to support the pleas of Florey and Chain for expanded production.

In America, in January 1942, the National Research Council formed a committee to organise clinical trials under the chairmanship of Dr. P. H. Long. The first trial, of staphylococcal infections, was arranged by Drs. Champ Lyons, C. S. Keefer, F. G. Blake, M. H. Dawson and W. Spink. During the same month of February, the firms of Merck and Squibb planned a collaborative effort and agreed to distribute information to other firms; all penicillin was to be supplied to and issued by the Committee on Medical Research. The first clinical test in America was carried out in March 1942. The patient was the wife of a Yale professor with puerperal infection and streptococcal septicaemia which had failed to respond to sulphanilamide. The penicillin, made by Merck, was given intravenously and cured the patient quickly. Between March and June enough penicillin was produced for systemic treatment of ten more patients. Thereafter production increased rapidly and about 200 cases were treated by the end of 1942, including 129 cases of gonorrhoea, among whom the success rate, as reported to the Committee, was 100%. The social impact of penicillin was beginning to be felt.

Up to this point, clinical trials in Britain had been arranged *ad hoc* by Florey. On September 25th, 1942 a General Penicillin Committee was formed to organise and co-ordinate further trials, and to regulate the use of the limited supplies. Small quantities of penicillin had already been used for the topical treatment of septic wounds in the desert army[21] and it was decided, in Britain and America, that future supplies should be used primarily for the armed forces. With production increasing rapidly, and further publications appearing[22-24], the virtues of penicillin were becoming widely known and the decision to restrict supplies to the armed forces caused resentment in some quarters. Each of the Services had to appoint its own area penicillin officers, who might or might not be experienced, to issue and supervise penicillin for therapy, with strict instructions not to release it for civilian use. It was said, correctly, that a soldier with a whitlow or gonorrhoea stood a much better chance of receiving penicillin than a civilian with septicaemia. Nevertheless, this restriction served a useful purpose. In the words of Florey and his colleagues[25], "It can be counted fortunate in this respect that the supplies of penicillin at the earliest stage of clinical application were so meagre, and the material so valuable, that a considerable degree of control could be maintained and a high standard of clinical work enforced. As a result, its mode of use was firmly based on facts which had been ascertained by experiment in the laboratory, thus ensuring within the limits of experience at that time the best use of the material in almost every case". Abuse was to follow, when rationing gave way to abundance.

Rapid as they were, therapeutic developments with penicillin were dependent entirely upon the volume of production. In the autumn of 1941, little or no penicillin for therapy was available in the United States. A year later, one firm supplied 1820 g to the Committee of Medical Research at a cost to the firm of $86,000, excluding overheads. In February 1943 the Office of Scientific Research and Development agreed to pay $200 per mega unit; this figure was dropped to $45 and then to $6 as production increased. In 1943 the main American producers were Merck, Squibb, Pfizer, Abbott, Winthrop and Commercial Solvents but, soon afterwards, eighteen firms were co-operating and four in Britain under terms which were designed to avoid giving advantage to any one company and to ensure reciprocal exchange of information between governmental, academic and industrial participants in the transatlantic programme. In the first six months of 1943, American production was about 400 million units; in the next six months, 20 billion units; by August 1945 production amounted to 650 billion units per month[26]. From a few selected centres designated for research and training in penicillin therapy in 1943, 2700 hospitals in the United States were so designated in January 1945. In Britain progress was much slower. This was partly due to shortage of facilities and finance, and to unavoidable war emergencies; but there were other difficulties, such as the failure to use submerged cultures and an unwillingness or inability in some quarters to recognise the unique properties of penicillin.

Quite apart from military considerations[27] and the relief of suffering, the knowledge gained by the rational use of penicillin between 1942 and 1946 in the American and British forces was incalculable. In the present day, when topical treatment with penicillin is discouraged and prophylaxis criticised, it is salutary to recall that thousands of lives were probably saved and innumerable disabilities prevented by these very methods during the campaigns in Normandy and elsewhere. It is hard for the post-penicillin era of doctors to realise that doses now regarded as inadequate (*e.g.* 15,000 units 4-hourly) were once employed successfully in the management of severe infections; and, more important, that many infections will resolve, completely and even beneficially, without any penicillin or other antibiotic being given. In contrast, when the body's defences were inadequate or when infection was massive, the benefits brought by penicillin when used properly were almost miraculous. By 1946 the conditions of use, dosage and standardisation of penicillin had been defined in all essentials, and supplies were adequate for civilian as well as military needs. In human affairs generally, tragedy and hardship are not infrequently due to failure to apply existing knowledge and to supply available materials. Penicillin is one supreme instance where no such failure was allowed to happen.

REFERENCES

[1] GOLDSWORTHY, N. E. AND FLOREY, H. W., *Brit. J. exp. Path.*, *11* (1930) 192.

[2] ROBERTS, E. A. H., *Quart. J. exp. Physiol.*, *27* (1937) 89.

[3] ABRAHAM, E. P., *Biochem. J.*, *33* (1938) 622.

[4] CLUTTERBUCK, P. W., LOVELL, R. AND RAISTRICK, H., *Biochem. J.*, *26* (1932) 1907.

[5] DOMAGK, G., *Dtsch. med. Wschr.*, 61, *250* (1935) 289.

[6] TRÉFOUEL, J., TRÉFOUEL, MME. J., NITTI, F. AND BOVET, D., *C.R. Soc. Biol. (Paris)*, *20* (1935) 756.

[7] HORLEIN, H., *Proc. roy. Soc. Med.*, *29* (1936) 313.

[8] COLEBROOK, L. AND KENNY, M., *Lancet, ii* (1936) 1319.

[9] CHAIN, E. B., FLOREY, H. W., GARDNER, A. D., HEATLEY, N. G. AND JENNINGS, M. A., *Lancet, ii* (1940) 177.

[10] HEATLEY, N. G., *Laboratory Practice, 10* (1961) 226.

[11] CHAIN, E. G., In FLOREY, *et al.*, *Antibiotics*, Vol. 2, Oxford University Press, 1949.

[12] CLARKE, H. T., JOHNSON, J. R. AND ROBINSON, R. (Eds.), *The Chemistry of the Penicillins*, Princeton University Press, 1949.

[13] ABRAHAM, E. P., CHAIN, E. B., FLETCHER, C. M., FLOREY, H. W., GARDNER, A. D., HEATLEY, N. G. AND JENNINGS, M. A., *Lancet, ii* (1941) 177.

14 FLEMING, A., *Pharm. J.*, *145* (1940) 172.
15 DAWSON, M. L., HOBBY, G. L., MEYER, K. AND CHAFFÉE, E., *J. clin. Invest.*, *20* (1941) 434.
16 COGHILL, R. D., *Chem. Eng. News*, *22* (1944) 588.
17 COGHILL, R. D. AND KOCH, R. S., *Chem. Eng. News*, *23* (1945) 2310.
18 FLOREY, M. E. AND FLOREY, H. W., *Lancet*, *i* (1943) 387.
19 CLARK, A. M., COLEBROOK, L., GIBSON, T., THOMSON, M. L. AND FOSTER, A., *Lancet*, *i* (1943) 605.
20 BODENHAM, D. C., *Lancet*, *ii* (1943) 725.
21 PULVERTAFT, R. J. V., *Lancet*, *ii* (1943) 341.
22 LYONS, C., *J. Amer. med. Assoc.*, *123* (1943) 1007.
23 KEEFER, C. S., BLAKE, F. G., MARSHALL, E. K., LOCKWOOD, J. S. AND WOOD, W. B., *J. Amer. med. Assoc.*, *122* (1943) 1217.
24 ANDERSON, D. G. AND KEEFER, C. S., *The therapeutic value of penicillin: treatment of 10,000 cases*, Edwards, Ann Arbor, (Mich.), 1948.
25 FLOREY, H. W., CHAIN, E., HEATLEY, N. G., JENNINGS, M. A., SANDERS, A. G., ABRAHAM, E. P. AND FLOREY, M. E., *Antibiotics*, Oxford University Press, 1949, p. 662.
26 RICHARDS, A. N., *Nature*, *201* (1964) 441.
27 See *History of Medical Research in the 2nd World War*, H.M.S.O., London, 1953.

Chapter 3

TWENTY YEARS LATER: THE NEW PENICILLINS

Rome lies gold and glad.

BROWNING

In many respects, penicillin was an ideal therapeutic substance, for it could be used with striking success prophylactically as well as therapeutically, combined high activity with negligible toxicity, and soon became cheap as well as easy to use. Since its chemical structure was soon known[1] and was comparatively simple, attempts at synthesis and modification of the molecule were obvious developments. It soon became known that antibacterial activity depended upon the nature of the side-chain. The nucleus (Fig. 2), consisting of a thiazolidine ring fused to a β-lactam ring, could only be formed at that time by biogenesis, presumably by an unusual cyclic fusion of the two constituent amino acids valine and cysteine. The final product however could be varied by adding different side-chain precursors to the culture fluid. Several forms of penicillin had been produced and systematically identified in this way. The highest degree of antibacterial activity resulted from the addition of phenylacetic acid which increased the yield of benzyl penicillin (penicillin G). Apart from its biogenesis by *Penicillium* spp., the β-lactam–thiazolidine ring structure was unknown in nature. Vigorous attempts at synthesis had been made by British and American scientists, working in close consultation during the war. Minute quantities of benzyl penicillin had actually been produced[2] by condensation of penicillamine with 2-benzyl-4-methoxymethylene-5(4)-oxazolone but, for practical purposes, synthesis by this route was unimportant. Sheehan and his colleagues in Boston described the synthesis of 5-phenyl penicillin[3] and two other β-lactam syntheses yielding substances with the chemical and physical properties of natural penicillins[4,5], but lacking in antibacterial activity.

Meanwhile, a clue that was to prove useful later came from Japan in 1950, when Sakaguchi and Murao[6] claimed that benzyl penicillin could be deacylated; three years later another Japanese worker, Kato[7] suggested that the intact β-lactam nucleus had thereby been liberated. These claims were probably correct but none of the Japanese scientists succeeded in isolating the nucleus. Using fermentative methods, Behrens *et al.*[8] succeeded in mak-

References p. 27/28

ing a phenoxymethyl side-chain which conferred acid stability upon the molecule. It was already known that *p*-hydroxyphenylacetic acid and other derivatives of acetic acid could be incorporated into the penicillin molecule by the mould biosynthetically. Several penicillins with substituted acetic acid side-chains were thereby produced[8]. These derivatives all possessed the antibacterial spectrum of penicillin G and were hydrolysed by penicillinase. Phenoxymethyl penicillin, was acid stable and was shown by Austrian workers[9] to be effective therapeutically. This was penicillin V, the first oral penicillin.

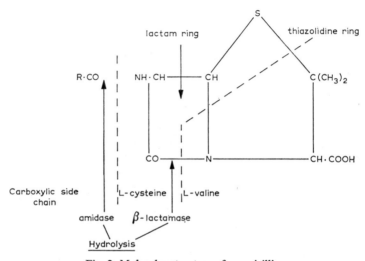

Fig. 2. Molecular structure of a penicillin.

The Boston group, under Sheehan, were continuing their attempts at total synthesis, encouraged by their success[10] in making a pure sulphonyl analogue of benzyl penicillin (benzenesulphonamidopenicillanic acid) which possessed some biological activity. The obstacle to synthesis was the cyclization of penicilloic acid to close the lactam ring of the nucleus (Fig. 3). After many trials and failures, Sheehan found that *N*-substituted carbodiimide reagents effected cyclization to form penicillin V from the corresponding penicilloic acid[11]. They also reported the presence of a key intermediate penicillinoate for the synthesis of further derivatives[12]. Production of these substances was however difficult; the yield was low and costly. Penicillin V was the only useful derivative and even this was easier to produce by biological methods. History was repeating itself at a higher biochemical level; for the second time the potentialities of penicillin were shortened by unique technical difficulties.

It was by this time abundantly clear what was required. An effective oral penicillin was now available but the antibacterial spectrum of penicillin V was narrower than that of penicillin G, and its intrinsic activity was lower. Resistant staphylococci had increased in prevalence and, with few exceptions, gram-negative bacilli were still outside the sphere of penicillin therapy. Sheehan had gone so far as to predict[13] in 1953 that the trend of chemical events would eventually produce penicillins which answered these problems

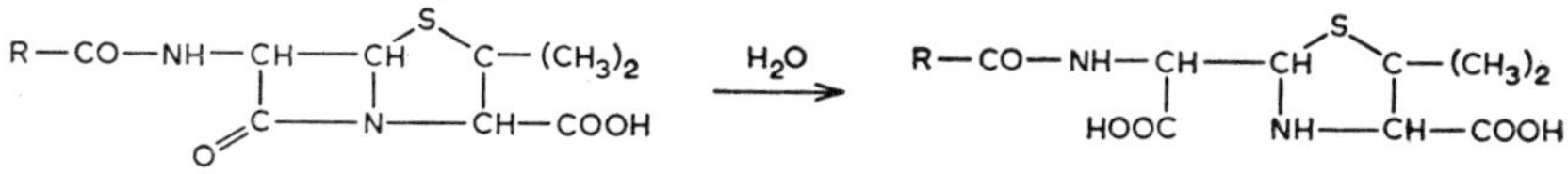

Fig. 3. Hydrolysis of penicillin to penicilloic acid.

by possessing (a) activity against resistant organisms, (b) wider spectrum, and (c) greater metabolic efficiency. His predictions were soon to be fulfilled from an unexpected quarter.

To those who live beyond its frontiers, scientific research is a cold, austere land where activities and relationships are impersonal. This is usually a myth and never more so than in the story of penicillin where fermentation characterised some of the personalities as well as the mould. At all the critical stages in this story there have been conflicts between imagination and earthiness, prospect and frustration.

The next major development was almost certainly a consequence of frustration. After the excellent teamwork which had been created during the war, first at Oxford and then on a transatlantic basis, Chain felt that much remained to be done and that the British effort and facilities should be enlarged. Like Fleming before him, but with more fire and eloquence and with the most remarkable collaborative achievement in medical science as his gospel, he attempted to persuade authorities that he stood at the entrance, not the exit, to research upon antibiotics. No one would have denied him the right, or modest facilities, to pursue his research; but, equally, no one in England with influence seems to have seen the need for a team. At Oxford, his erstwhile colleagues preferred to continue their researches on academic lines; at St. Mary's, there was no space and little opportunity; industry concentrated, profitably enough, upon the production of penicillin G by American methods. Chain saw that, in this field of research, accomplishment was the fusion of academic exploration with industrial gearing; he wanted a research laboratory with a pilot plant beside it, manned by biochemists, microbiologists, chemical engineers and other specialists, who could pool their expertise. To those in authority in post-war Britain, this sounded like a romantic dream; to the finance committees, like a hideous nightmare. With both authorities against him, he accepted an invitation from the Institute of Public Health of the Italian State to organise a biochemical and micro-biological department, with its own pilot plant, at Rome.

In most countries, penicillin became available for general use between 1945 and 1950. It was used widely, but not always wisely, and some complications began to occur. In some countries it was sold over the counter to the general public in the form of skin cream, nasal ointment, lozenges and other popular medicaments; even where its use was restricted, as in Great Britain, it was often prescribed for cutaneous infections and applied topically. Since penicillin can be allergenic (see Chapter 14), its usage in this fashion induced hypersensitivity in many people, especially those who subsequently received it parenterally. When lozenges were used, the sensitive coccal flora of the pharynx was suppressed and replaced by resistant organisms including coliforms and *Candida albicans*; sometimes a troublesome stomatitis developed. Reports of these and other complications appeared increasingly in the medical press and soon led, in most countries, to legislation restricting the sale of penicillin-containing medicaments. The topical application of penicillin by physicians gradually lost acceptance as a therapeutic procedure. Some of these problems were therefore self-limiting, but not before many patients had been highly and dangerously sensitised to penicillin. A relatively high proportion of hypersensitive subjects seen today acquired their idiosyncrasy from topical applications in these early days. At the same time it should be remembered that a great deal of infection was probably eliminated in the process. Drug-resistance also began to emerge on a major scale during this period though, from the practical viewpoint, this problem was confined to staphylococci. The origin and evolution of these organisms, in the earliest stages, is unexplained through lack of statistical data. It is known that some strains of staphylococci were relatively resistant to penicillin *ab initio*[14] but their prevalence is uncertain. Fleming's early records make no mention of any staphylococcus being resistant, but his methods were perhaps insufficiently quantitative to reveal this. The Oxford workers in 1940 regarded staphylococci as being sensitive though, from the start, their assays were quantitative and they were well aware of the widely-differing sensitivities of the main pathogenic bacteria. From that point onward, penicillin began to be used therapeutically and most hospitals interested in assay of routine isolates were also embarking upon therapy. It is clear however that, in the case of *Staph. aureus*, sensitive strains do not acquire resistance during therapy; this conclusion was drawn from therapeutic results at an early date, before the intricacies of penicillinase production had been studied, but it is none the less still true. The resistant strains which began to be described in 1945 and thereafter were penicillinase formers which spread to hospitals by cross-infection[15-17]. By 1950 the spread was beginning to be uncontrollable.

The position of penicillin in the 1950's was therefore less satisfactory than in 1945, despite great refinements in manufacture and world-wide production on a scale which had lowered the price well below that of any other antibiotic. But price and supply were not the problems. To maintain and extend the control of bacterial infection, a fresh approach was needed.

Among the firms interested in the potential of antibiotic research during the war was the Beecham group of companies, well known for proprietary medicines, toilet preparations and patent foods, but not at all known for ethical pharmaceutical products. Penicillin production at that time was under the Ministry of Supply, which refused a licence. The company retained its interest with lowered sights and received in 1945 a contract from the Air Ministry for making penicillin pastilles. Their deeper purpose was to enter the field of ethical products and to conduct research. For this purpose a large house was acquired at Brockham Park in Surrey for conversion into research laboratories, and opened by Sir Alexander Fleming on 18th June, 1947. By 1952, with a new and energetic chairman, Mr. H. G. Lazell, these laboratories were handling several projects under the direction of Dr. John Farquharson, including the synthesis of amino acids and small peptides, and were attempting the stabilisation of penicillin G for oral use by various buffered formulations. The marketing of penicillin V in 1954 led to the cancellation of attempts to produce an oral penicillin G and to a reappraisal of the firm's position in antibiotic research. On the advice of Sir Charles Dodds, an approach was made to Professor E. B. Chain, in Rome, for further guidance and collaboration in this regard. It will be recalled that Chain had gone to Rome to fulfil his plan of including a miniature industrial plant in his research laboratory. He agreed with the Beecham representatives and advisers (Sir Ian Heilbron and Dr. A. H. Cook) that there was room and opportunity for further research on antibiotics and suggested, specifically, that they should pursue (*a*) molecular modifications leading toward penicillinase-stable and broad-spectrum penicillins, and (*b*) new mutants of the mould. He agreed to collaborate along these lines and, with the agreement of the Director, Professor Marotta, arrangements were made for the work to be started at Chain's laboratories in the Istituto Superiore di Sanità. Meanwhile, the Beecham team was strengthened by the recruitment of Dr. G. N. Rolinson, a microbiologist, and Mr. F. Batchelor, a biochemist. The new recruits went to Rome to begin work at the beginning of 1956; meanwhile, microbiological laboratories were being built at Brockham Park, where the chemistry department, under Mr. F. P. Doyle and Dr. J. H. C. Nayler, was already active in the preparation of penicillin precursors for the company now known as Beecham Research Laboratories Ltd.

At Chain's suggestion, the research team at Rome began work on the biosynthesis of *p*-aminobenzyl penicillin[18] with the collaboration of Dr. A. Ballio and Dr. Dentice di Accadia of the Istituto's staff. It was hoped that the reactive NH_2 group on this derivative would provide a point of attachment for additional side-chains. By adding *p*-aminophenylacetic acid as precursor to the fermentation flasks, the *p*-aminobenzyl derivative was produced to the extent of about 40% of the total penicillin activity. This fermentation was transferred from the flasks to the 50-litre fermentation vats in Chain's laboratory and, by October 1956, only nine months after beginning work, reasonable quantities of the derivative, 80% pure, were available from each fermentation[19]. Meanwhile, the microbiological laboratories and plant had been completed at Brockham Park, whither the Beecham workers returned. The research team at Brockham Park consisted essentially of J. Farquharson (Director), G. N. Rolinson (Fermentation and microbiology), F. R. Batchelor (Biochemistry), F. P. Doyle and J. H. C. Nayler (Chemistry), M. Richards (Mycology), D. M. Brown and P. Acred (Pharmacology), G. C. Eustace (Pilot plant), with the assistance of Miss S. Stevens (Microbiological assay) and Messrs. Pillow, Soulal, Stove and Willcox (Chemistry and Development). Having planned to enter the field of fundamental research upon and development of penicillin on 18th May, 1955, the Beecham group was by effort alone in a strong position to implement its intentions by January, 1957 with the facilities developed at Brockham Park. Then luck lent a hand.

Until this stage, modification of the penicillin molecule had been attempted essentially by the precursor route, ever since it had been found that the addition of phenylacetic acid or its amide increased the yield of benzyl penicillin in fermentation. Prior to 1952, some few hundred penicillins had been made by adding different precursors, though the only one of real value was phenoxymethyl penicillin (V). In most laboratories, the products of fermentation were assayed, as a routine, by chemical as well as microbiological methods. It was well-known that discrepancies often occurred between the two, and in some laboratories a correction factor to allow for this discrepancy was regularly applied. The chemical method, usually performed by adding hydroxylamine which reacted with the penicillin to give a hydroxamic acid, usually gave a higher value than microbiological assay of active penicillin. It was noticed in Rome and subsequently that the discrepancy was larger when no precursor was added. They had not at that time read the Japanese report by Kato[7] but it was clear that there was a substance present in the fermentation liquor which had the properties of a penicillin in that it reacted with hydroxylamine and was destroyed by penicillinase and yet lacked the full antibacterial activity of a penicillin. This substance must be either an inactive penicillin or the nucleus of 6-aminopenicillanic acid (6-APA). The suggestion was then made—so casually that no one remembers who made it—that, if the inactive substance was 6-APA, acetylation should yield benzylpenicillin. This was done by adding phenylacetyl chloride (Fig. 4)

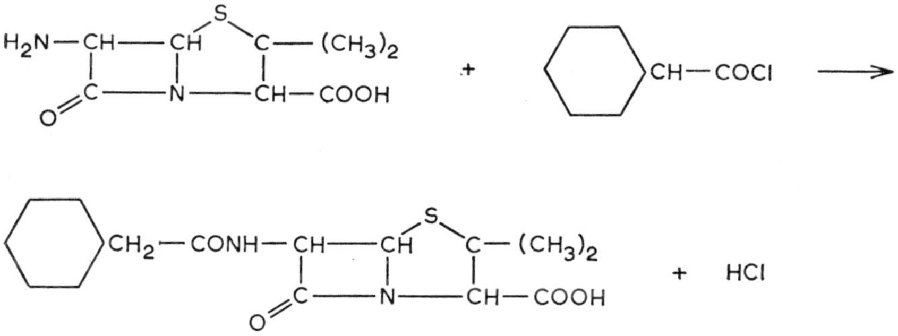

Fig. 4. Phenylacetylation of 6-APA.

and the resulting product was indeed benzylpenicillin[21]. The news of this experiment in May 1957 was immediately conveyed to Dr. Farquharson, who ordered that all other work should cease while this experiment was reinvestigated thoroughly and repeated. The technique of paper chromatography and bioassay of the strips[21] was used intensively for this purpose and, in June 1957, the results were amply confirmed and documented. The implication of this finding was that, if pure 6-APA could be isolated, the possibilities for altering the activity of penicillin by adding new side-chains in the 6-position were immense. At a meeting in July 1957 it was agreed that the

References p. 27/28

progamme on p-aminobenzyl penicillin should cease and that work on the isolation and modification of 6-APA should take precedence over all other research activities.

Intelligent observation, good luck and a keen follow-up had cleared the way for a rapid advance. But some difficulties still stood in the path. 6-APA was amphoteric and hydrophilic, so that it could not be extracted from the fermentation liquor by organic solvents; it was unstable to heat and in solution; its solubility was extremely low at the isoelectric point. The yield was therefore low, only about 20 g in 10–14 days from 400 l of fermented medium. By January 1958 however pure 6-APA had been prepared by a complicated extraction procedure. By this stage the Japanese work had been read and it became apparent that a fermentation mould could yield an enzyme capable of yielding 6-APA by deacylation of preformed penicillins. This indicated the opening to a new and easier avenue for the preparation of 6-APA, and various fungi were therefore investigated for acylase activity. Among other organisms which were found to produce this type of enzyme, *Streptomyces lavendulae* formed an exocellular amidase which readily reacylated penicillin V[22]. As a result of this process, the yield of 6-APA was increased so that the preparation of derivatives became easier. By the end of 1958, many new derivatives were being examined. At this stage, with patent applications lodged, papers reporting these results were drafted for *Nature*[21,22] and other journals[23,24].

Before the commencement of the programme of biosynthesis of new penicillins, Beecham Research Laboratories had engaged in negotiations with the American company Bristol–Myers about the possibility of collaborative work on penicillins. No definite arrangements had been made but, early in 1959, the Beecham group informed the Bristol Company of their recent findings and invited their co-operation in the production of new derivatives of 6-APA. Bristol accepted this invitation and a short-term agreement was signed for collaboration in research, development and production. After the first papers by the Beecham group had appeared in *Nature* (17th and 24th January, 1959) a press conference was held; on the following day (7th March) the *Lancet* commented upon the importance of these developments in an annotation though, a week later, the *British Medical Journal* voiced some doubt (p. 701). In June, representatives of the Bristol Company visited Brockham Park, accompanied by Professor John Sheehan, of the Massachusetts Institute of Technology, as adviser (see p. 18). In the work that followed, Bristol made 6-APA by fermentation, Beecham by enzymatic hydrolysis of penicillins G or V.

By this time, Beechams had prepared several hundred derivatives and some important basic facts were being established.

(*1*) 6-APA, though lacking the activity of benzyl penicillin against gram-positive organisms, retained more or less equivalent activity against gram-negative bacilli.

(*2*) The α-carbon atom of the side-chain proved to be a key location for substituents.

(*3*) Substitution of the "hindered acid" triphenylacetic acid in place of phenylacetic acid conferred stability to penicillinase and gave rise later to the concept of steric hindrance at the site of attachment of this enzyme.

Fact (*1*) foreshadowed the development of penicillins active against gram-negative bacilli, though this possibility had already been glimpsed in the activity of substances like *p*-aminobenzyl penicillin and cephalosporin N (see p. 106). Fact (*2*) led to the preparation of more acid-stable penicillins by the introduction of methyl or other groups in the α-position. Fact (*3*) led to the preparation of methicillin. The era of systematic biosynthesis in the chemotherapy of infection was being born.

The first derivative prepared for clinical trial and marketing was the acid-stable α-phenoxymethyl penicillin, 6-(α-phenoxypropionamido)-penicillanic acid. The potassium salt of this acid was highly soluble; the phenoxy group ensured acid stability and the presence of the additional methyl group in the α-position conferred better absorption than penicillin V. This compound, developed by Bristol more than by Beechams, though known to both groups, was marketed in the United States and United Kingdom in November 1959 after a brief clinical trial[25–27]. With the official name phenethicillin, it was the forerunner of a short series of acid-stable derivatives possessing similar properties. The therapeutic advantages of these compounds (see p. 33) were and are hypothetical, depending entirely upon improved absorption at the expense of intrinsic antibacterial activity. In scientific medical circles, the advent of phenethicillin as the first offspring of the new biosyntheses was something of an anticlimax and the reception was correspondingly luke-warm. With Expectation in the air, as well as in the scientific press, better things had been awaited.

Fortunately, developments of deeper significance were in hand. Derivative 1060, produced at Brockham Park, was a mixture of two epimers with amino groups attached to the α-carbon of phenylacetic acid. This compound was therefore acid stable and also possessed enhanced activity against gram-negative bacilli. While this substance was being investigated, a compound of greater immediate interest (BRL 1241) was made, and BRL 1060 was almost discarded. At a later date, however, after some clinical and further experimental work, BRL 1060 was salvaged to widen the scope of penicillin therapy (Chapter 6).

During this time, the attractive hypothesis of steric hindrance of the side-chain had gripped the attention of the young research team at Brockham Park. The triphenylmethyl derivative of 6-APA (compound 1071) looked interesting, for it was stable in the presence of penicillinase while yet possessing antibacterial activity. When tested in animals, however, it was so highly protein–bound that it remained at the site of injection. Among other hindered substances tested was 2,6-dimethoxybenzoic acid whose acid chloride reacted directly with 6-APA to give an acid whose sodium salt 6-(2,6-dimethoxybenzamido) penicillanate monohydrate, Compound 1241, showed a combination of useful properties: activity against gram-positive cocci; stability to penicillinase; high aqueous solubility; non-toxicity in animals. Clinical trials followed and the drug now known as methicillin was marketed simultaneously in the United States and United Kingdom along with the first published reports in the *British Medical Journal* of 3rd September 1960. This drug, arriving at a time when the menace of the resistant hospital staphylococcus was at its height, was widely welcomed. A curious problem arose over its classification: by definition, a penicillin had to be a substance hydrolysed by penicillinase and for an amusing moment it was questionable whether this much-needed penicillin could be classified as such!

The year 1961 saw further work, mainly in America, on the preparation of additional acid-stable α-phenoxymethyl derivatives. This led to the marketing of propicillin and other compounds with theoretical advantages over penicillin V. Two more important developments also occurred, however. In Britain, D(—) 6-(α-aminophenylacetamido)-penicillanic acid, BRL 1341, was identified as the more active epimer of compound 1060, and tried clinically in patients with gram-negative infections. This led to the marketing of ampicillin in the summer of 1961. In America, the Bristol group had concentrated upon the isoxazolyl derivatives of 6-APA which had been synthesised at Brockham Park and were stable to both acid and penicillinase. Bristol selected for clinical trial the parent derivative 5-methyl-3-phenyl-4-isoxazolyl penicillin, but Beechams and their advisers preferred, for various reasons (p. 40), the halogenated derivatives, in particular compound 1621 with a chlorine atom in the 5-position on the benzene ring. Both drugs have now been marketed for the oral treatment of infections due to penicillinase-forming staphylococci. Theoretically, any number of side-chains can be added to the 6-APA molecule and it is conceivable that modification of the nucleus itself may also be accomplished. It is likely therefore that in the next few years a number of derivatives will be produced, though it may be timely now to urge caution. The older penicillins and the new derivatives at present in use seem to possess in common the most important single characteristic of the penicillins, that is, lack of toxicity. With increasing complexity of the side-chain, this attribute might be lost. There is a need now for consolidation of existing gains coupled with a more exacting scrutiny of any new derivatives.

Whereas the development of penicillin G was inevitably a mammoth effort involving many departments in Government, Universities, hospitals and many industrial firms, that of the semisynthetic penicillins was a quiet and unofficial affair, confined to a handful of scientists, two industrial plants and a few hospitals. The problems and targets were much smaller but, even so, the pace and pattern of advance are exemplary. The story is a minor classic of the circumstances which engender scientific progress: the sound plan for research, the competent all-round team, the probing of a significant anomaly, the good idea, the quick exploitation, and, by no means least, the moral and material support of management and advisers. As with penicillin G, it is a story of purposeful team work between industry, hospitals and academic departments, and it is a story worth repeating, for there has been no better road as yet to the cure of disease by medicine.

REFERENCES

[1] CLARKE, H. T., JOHNSON, J. R. AND ROBINSON, R. (Eds.), *Chemistry of Penicillin*, Princeton University Press, 1949.
[2] FOLKERS, K. In TODD, A. (Ed.), *Perspectives in Organic Chemistry*, Interscience, New York, 1956.
[3] SHEEHAN, J. C., BUHLE, E. L., COREY, E. J., LAUBACH, G. D. AND RYAN, J. J., *J. Amer. chem. Soc.*, 72 (1950) 3828.
[4] SHEEHAN, J. C. AND IZZO, P. T., *J. Amer. chem. Soc.*, 71 (1949) 4059.
[5] SHEEHAN, J. C. AND BOSE, A. K., *J. Amer. chem. Soc.*, 72 (1950) 5158.
[6] SAKAGUCHI, K. AND MURAO, S., *J. agric. chem. Soc. Japan*, 23 (1950) 411.
[7] KATO, K., *J. Antibiot. (Tokyo)*, A6, 130 (1953) 184.
[8] BEHRENS, O. K., CORSE, J., EDWARDS, J. P., GARRISON, L. L., JONES, R. G., SOPER, Q. F. VAN ABEELE, F. R. AND WHITEHEAD, C. W., *J. biol. Chem.*, 175 (1948) 793.
[9] BRANDL, E., GIOVANNINI, M. AND MARGREITER, H., *Wien. med. Wschr.*, 103 (1953) 602.
[10] SHEEHAN, J. C. AND HOFF, D. R., *J. Amer. chem. Soc.*, 79 (1957) 1262.
[11] SHEEHAN, J. C. AND HENERY-LOGAN, K. R., *J. Amer. chem. Soc.*, 79 (1957) 1262.
[12] SHEEHAN, J. C. AND HENERY-LOGAN, K. R., *J. Amer. chem. Soc.*, 81 (1958) 3089.
[13] SHEEHAN, J. C., *Meeting of the American Chemical Society, Ann Arbor (Mich)*, 1953.
[14] KIRBY, W. M. M., *Science*, 99 (1944) 452.

[15] BONDI, A. AND DIETZ, C. C., *Proc. Soc. exp. Biol.*, *60* (1945) 55.
[16] KIRBY, W. M. M., *J. clin. Invest.*, *24* (1945) 165.
[17] BARBER, M., *J. Path. Bact.*, *59* (1947) 373.
[18] CORSE, J. W., JONES, R. G., SOPER, Q. F., WHITEHEAD, C. W. AND BEHRENS, O. K., *J. Amer. chem. Soc.*, *70* (1948) 2837.
[19] BALLIO, A., CHAIN, E. B., DENTICE DI ACCADIA, F., BATCHELOR, F. R. AND ROLINSON, G. N., *Nature*, *183* (1959) 180.
[20] MURAO, S., *J. agric. chem. Soc. Japan*, *29* (1955) 400, 404.
[21] BATCHELOR, F. R., DOYLE, F. P., NAYLER, J. H. C. AND ROLINSON, G. N., *Nature*, *183* (1959) 257.
[22] ROLINSON, G. N., BATCHELOR, F. R., BUTTERWORTH, D., CAMERON-WOOD, J., COLE, M., EUSTACE, G. C., MART, MARIAN V., RICHARDS, M. AND CHAIN, E. B., *Nature*, *187* (1960) 236.
[23] BATCHELOR, F. R., CHAIN, E. B., AND ROLINSON, G. N., *Proc. roy. Soc. B, 154* (1961) 478.
[24] BATCHELOR, F. R., CHAIN, E. B., HARDY, T. L., MANSFORD, K. R. L. AND ROLINSON, G. N., *Proc. roy. Soc. B, 154* (1961) 498.
[25] MORIGI, E. M. E., WHEATLEY, W. B. AND ALBRIGHT, H., *Antibiot. Ann.*, 1959–60 (1959). 127.
[26] CRONK, G. A., NAUMANN, D. E., ALBRIGHT, H. AND WHEATLEY, W. B., *Antibiot. Ann.*, 1959–60 (1959) 133.
[27] KNUDSEN, E. T. AND ROLINSON, G. N., *Lancet, ii* (1959) 1105.

Chapter 4

ACID-STABLE PENICILLINS. I

GENERAL CONSIDERATIONS; PHENOXYMETHYL DERIVATIVES

The advent of the new penicillins caused an upheaval of established therapeutic procedures and policies, especially in hospitals. With the menace of staphylococcal cross-infection controllable if not controlled, there was less need to keep antibiotics like erythromycin in reserve or to devise rotations and combinations of antibiotics designed to minimise drug resistance. In the words of an American writer[1], penicillins are again "the agents of choice for all gram-positive coccic infections". In addition, the introduction of ampicillin gives them a place in the treatment of many infections due to gram-negative bacilli.

On grounds of lack of toxicity and convenience of administration, the oral penicillins are agents of first choice in a variety of infections. There are however important differences between these drugs, which are seldom mutually interchangeable (Table I). Ampicillin has the widest range of activity by far, but is inactive against penicillinase-forming organisms including resistant staphylococci. At the other extreme, the isoxazole penicillins and nafcillin are highly active against penicillinase-forming staphylococci and certain other pyogenic cocci, but virtually inactive against everything else. Between these extremes come the four phenoxy penicillins which have paradoxical antibacterial and pharmacological properties: as the aliphatic chain lengthens antibacterial activity diminishes and narrows, but alimentary absorption improves. The position has therefore been reached when plasma levels two or three times as high as those of penicillin V can be produced by drugs with one-half to one-third of its activity. Whether or not this is an advantage remains to be seen. Higher plasma levels may permit diffusion of these drugs into relatively inaccessible situations like the middle ear, but this has not yet been proved and, even if it occurs, can only be of benefit against a limited range of sensitive organisms. Finland and his colleagues[2,3] have attempted to rationalise this problem by testing the antibacterial power of the serum after doses of different phenoxy penicillins; such studies[4] suggest that penicillin V is equal or superior to the other derivatives. There are few controlled clinical trials comparing these drugs[5] but there is some evidence[6,7]

References p. 36/37

TABLE I

ACID-STABLE ORAL PENICILLINS

Side-chain	Official name	Activity against				Limitations
		Staphy-lococcus	P-ase staphy-lococcus	Other cocci	Gram-negative bacilli	
6-(phenoxyacetamido)-	Penicillin V	High	Nil	High	Nil	Variable absorption
6-(α-phenoxypropion-amido)-	Phenethicillin	High	Low	Variable	Nil	Less active than penicillin V against streptococci and pneumococci
6-(α-phenoxybutyr-amido)-	Propicillin	High	Low	Variable	Nil	
6-(α-phenoxyphenyl-acetamido)-	Phenbenicillin	High	Low	Variable	Nil	
6-(5-methyl-3-phenyl-4-isoxazole-carboxamido)-	Oxacillin	High	High	Variable	Nil	Variable absorption Narrow spectrum
6-(5-methyl-3-orthochlorophenyl-4-isoxazole-carboxamido)-	Cloxacillin	High	High	Medium	Nil	Narrow spectrum
6-(2-ethoxy-1-naphthamido)-	Nafcillin	High	High	Variable	Nil	Variable absorption Narrow spectrum
6-(D(−)-α-amino-phenylacetamido)-	Ampicillin	High	Nil	High	Medium	Gram-negative bacilli may become resistant during therapy

that blood concentrations are more easily maintained with the longer-chain derivatives; it has also been claimed[8,9] that phenethicillin is marginally more effective than penicillin V in the treatment of streptococcal otitis media.

AVAILABLE FORMS OF ACID-STABLE PENICILLINS

6-(phenoxyacetamido)-penicillanic acid
(phenoxymethyl penicillin or penicillin V, potassium salt)

The first steps in the production of penicillin V, by modification of the fermentative process, were made[10] in 1948. The therapeutic implications were not immediately realised and it was not until 1953 that penicillin V came into

clinical use[11,12]. Early hopes that it would be an oral replacement for penicillin G were soon dashed by more critical microbiological tests which showed
(ref. 13) that it was relatively inactive against the gonococcus, haemophilus
and other gram-negative organisms. The presence of a polar group in the
side-chain, however, conferred acid stability upon an active penicillin for the
first time and set the pattern for subsequent molecular modifications.

Penicillin V is most active when used in the form of the potassium salt.
Absorption begins 1.5–2 h after oral administration, according to the state
of fullness and motility of the stomach, producing with standard doses
(250–500 mg in an adult) plasma levels of 3–4 $\mu g/ml$. Excretion, mainly in
the urine, occurs rapidly but is by no means quantitative[14]. This may be due
to incomplete absorption or to destruction in the gut, for this form of penicillin is susceptible to the action of inactivating enzymes (see p. 142). The
peak plasma concentration, and hence the diffusion potential, is higher
when it is given to the patient fasting, but the same total amount is absorbed
if it is taken with or after meals. In terms of activity, 60 mg of penicillin V is
roughly equal to 100,000 units of penicillin G.

Between 1953 and 1959, penicillin V was the only reliable oral penicillin
and was therefore very widely used. It was found to be reliable in the treatment of many common infections[15] due to gram-positive cocci, especially
streptococci of group A and pneumococci; it was therefore valuable in
treating pharyngitis and in preventing or treating complications of upper
respiratory infections such as sinusitis and otitis media. As with other oral
penicillins, its efficacy depends largely upon its being given in the early
stages of infection when the infected site is hyperaemic; when lesions are
more deep-seated, as in established otitis media, pneumonia and empyema,
it is much less reliable. In these circumstances it is wise to begin treatment
with one or more injections of penicillin G intramuscularly and to use
penicillin V for continuation of therapy. Even in large doses it is unsuitable
for the treatment of any form of meningitis. American workers[16] claimed
that doses of 4–6 g daily are effective in maintaining control of some cases of
subacute bacterial endocarditis. Prolonged therapy on this scale changes the
bacterial flora of the gut and oropharynx and it is advisable to watch for
side-effects like superinfection with *Candida albicans* and other organisms,
stomatitis and perineal pruritis.

Prophylactic use of penicillin V

One of the major uses of penicillin V is the chemoprophylaxis of streptococcal infection in patients who are subject to rheumatic fever or glomerulo-

References p. 36/37

nephritis. For this purpose, low doses are usually deemed to be sufficient[17,18] and can be continued for months or years, usually without side-effects except for the occasional development of hypersensitivity[18]. Some authorities allege that "a mere whiff of penicillin is enough to keep the highly sensitive haemolytic streptococcus away"[19], but the dose must not be too low. Cope and his colleagues[20] found that 60 mg twice daily was incompletely effective: only one case acquired a group A streptococcus and there was no tonsillitis in 25 rheumatic subjects during 3 years of close surveillance, but the antistreptolysin O titre rose in several patients. Penicillin V was superior to penicillin G (200,000 units orally twice daily) which is sometimes recommended, but is was considered that 240 mg should be given twice daily. On the other hand, there are hazards in continuing such relatively high dosage over a long period: for instance, Harris et al.[21] found a 48% incidence of superinfection by penicillin-resistant staphylococci, with two fatalities, in a group of children. This kind of incidence is probably influenced by environmental factors as well as dosage, for some workers[22] found no major changes in the flora of the throat during long-term prophylaxis. Nevertheless, the possibility of superinfection is sometimes high and additional measures, such as antibacterial nasal cream and frequent swabbing, may be required if intensive prophylaxis is to be conducted with safety, in outpatients as well as in closed communities. The most serious superinfections are those due to *Staph. aureus*, usually group III strains, for the carriage-rate in the throat rises sharply during prophylaxis, and other drugs may be required to eradicate these organisms; if they persist, the usual alternative is to change to sulphonamide prophylaxis, which is more toxic and less effective[17]. Other organisms may also colonise the oropharynx: coliforms are common and can usually be disregarded except in infants or debilitated patients. *Candida albicans* is not uncommon and can also be disregarded in the absence of lesions, or if present only in cultures. Stomatitis due to this or other organisms necessitates a temporary withdrawal of oral prophylaxis while the lesions are treated by appropriate topical or other measures.

Apart from these disadvantages, which are seldom serious, prolonged chemoprophylaxis is a well-established and successful practice for the prevention of recurrence of rheumatic fever, especially in children, and penicillin V is at present the drug of choice for this purpose. The other acid-stable penicillins may be suitable as alternatives but seem to offer no obvious advantages unless staphylococcal superinfection occurs, in which event cloxacillin may be useful, though as yet unproved.

As an indication of the results of continuous chemoprophylaxis over a long period, the findings of RuDusky[23] are of interest. Among military recruits in the U.S.A. examined during the period 1941–1963, there was a 63% decrease in rheumatic heart disease, and this was attributed primarily to the use of antibacterial drugs during the period. Of those with valvular heart disease, only 7% were under chemoprophylaxis. It should be remembered that the incidence of rheumatic fever has also decreased during this period, almost to the point of rarity. The role of penicillin in this decrease cannot be assessed statistically, but circumstantial evidence points strongly to its importance (see p. 173).

Penicillin V or other oral penicillins can also be used prophylactically during dental extractions, tonsillectomy and other surgical procedures to lessen the risk of streptococcal infection in patients with valvular disease of the heart or nephritis. With the exception of ampicillin, the oral penicillins are not suitable for preventing exacerbations in chronic bronchitis, on account of their narrow antibacterial spectra.

6-(α-phenoxypropionamido)-penicillanic acid (Phenethicillin)

This was the first substance produced biosynthetically from 6-APA with enough biological activity to warrant therapeutic trial in 1959. Molecularly it was modelled upon penicillin V, since it was known that the introduction of a phenoxy group conferred acid stability. At equivalent doses, the potassium salt was found by Knudsen and Rolinson[24] to be better absorbed though the reasons for this are still not clear. Like the other longer-chain phenoxy derivatives, it is less susceptible than penicillins G and V to inactivating enzymes (see p. 142). The unchanged drug is rapidly excreted to the extent of 60% of the ingested dose, but not all of it is unchanged, for a metabolite is formed in the body (p. 126).

The main promise of phenethicillin and, indeed, of the other phenoxy-derivatives described below, lay in improved absorption. Critical microbiology[13,25] showed it to be much less active than penicillins G or V against pyogenic cocci, and narrower in spectrum; it was also more highly protein bound[26] and this appeared to interfere with its antibacterial activity, as assessed in vitro. To investigate these factors, Jackson et al.[27] measured the bactericidal effect of phenethicillin, compared with penicillins G and V, on Streptococcus viridans at defined stages in the presence of varying amounts of serum. They found that the presence of protein did not always interfere with bactericidal action; for instance, low concentrations (10%) interfered with phenethicillin more than with the other penicillins, whereas neat serum (100%) did the reverse. From these experiments and from clinical studies conducted in parallel, they concluded that phenethicillin was as effective as the other penicillins in eradicating streptococci causing endocarditis. A subsequent study[28] from the same centre in Chicago indicated that endocarditis caused by certain sensitive strains of streptococci could be cured. The strains were all α-haemolytic and phenethicillin was bactericidal in the presence of serum in concentrations of about 0.12 μg/ml. Dosage at the rate of 0.5–1.0 g every 4 h in adults produced peak serum levels of 4–32 μg/ml at 1–1.5 h, falling to 0.06–16 μg/ml at 3–4.5 h. Probenecid (0.5 g every 6 h) was given to the patients with lower serum levels, with good effect.

These results, in an infection which is notoriously difficult to treat, suggest strongly that the effect of phenethicillin depends mainly upon the serum concentration attained. If the organism is sensitive and if a bactericidal concentration of drug is reached and maintained, the organism will be eradicated despite the supposed interference of protein binding. Judged by this token, simpler infections should be easier to treat and it would appear that, with proper dosage of 20–40 mg/kg/day, streptococci of group A and pneumococci should be within the range of the drug. It should be remembered however that, due to variability in absorption or other factors, oral penicillins may wholly fail to control severe infections such as pneumonia, mastoiditis and meningitis. The writer recently saw a child aged 3 years who had developed pneumococcal meningitis while receiving full doses of phenethicillin.

As prepared at present, phenethicillin is a racemic mixture containing 55–75% of the L-isomer and 25–45% of the D-isomer. It was originally claimed[29] that the mixture was more active than either component but subsequent studies do not support this claim. Finland and his colleagues[30,31] showed that L-phenethicillin, or the mixture, was more active against gram-positive organisms *in vitro* than the D-isomer. English and McBride[32] found the L-isomer more effective against staphylococcal infection in mice, and Cronk et al.[33] reported that higher blood levels were obtained when this isomer was given to human subjects. From these studies, the L-isomer is clearly more active though, for reasons not yet explained, the DL mixture often appears to be equally active. The relative proportions of each isomer required to give this effect are unknown. It is therefore clearly desirable that, in any preparation issued for therapeutic use, an adequate amount of the L-isomer should be present and that the reasons for these differences in biological activity of the isomers should be explored.

6-(α-phenoxybutyramido)-penicillanic acid
(α-phenoxypropyl penicillin, Propicillin)

This substance is the third analogue in the phenoxymethyl (penicillin V) group of derivatives of 6-APA. Used as the potassium salt of a mixture of two optically-active isomers, it is readily soluble in water and acid stable.

Propicillin has the narrow antibacterial spectrum of phenethicillin; its intrinsic activity against the pyogenic cocci is of a similar order or lower. When given orally, it is well-absorbed, giving peak levels in about 1 h, which are much higher than those given by equivalent doses of penicillin V and slightly higher than thoses of phenethicillin[33].

Like phenethicillin, propicillin is more active than penicillin V against penicillinase-forming staphylococci[34,35]. This does not mean that these organisms as a class can be classified as "sensitive" to this kind of penicillin, but it is possible that the marginal increase in activity thus signified might lessen the tendency toward staphylococcal superinfection during therapy. According to one report[36] propicillin is effective in eradicating staphylococci from the sputum in patients with respiratory infections.

6-(α-phenoxyphenylacetamido)-penicillanic acid
(Phenbenicillin, the potassium salt)

The acid stability and antibacterial range of this soluble salt are very similar to those of phenethicillin. It is essentially a narrow spectrum substance and its only importance is the high and sustained plasma concentration after oral dosage. Thus Rollo *et al.*[37] found in 18 subjects a mean level of about 5 μg/ml 0.5 and 1 h after a dose of 150 mg, compared with 1.6 and 1 μg/ml with penicillin V and 2 and 1.6 with phenethicillin; after 4–6 h, residual levels with phenbenicillin were higher than with the other two drugs which were, more often than not, undetectable. It is claimed that doses of 125 mg give higher peak values, persisting longer than double the dose of penicillin V. Urinary excretion is lower than with other penicillins, only 20–25% of a given dose being excreted; part of this—about one-fifth— consists of two active metabolites of unknown structure, the remainder being unchanged drug. Toxicity to animals is very low and the drug appears to be well-tolerated in human subjects, though data is scanty as yet.

In a clinical study, Carter and Brumfitt[38] found that a variety of streptococcal, pneumococcal and staphylococcal infections (penicillin-sensitive) responded "promptly". Most of these 20 cases had relatively minor infections and only one relapsed—a pyosalpinx due to an anaerobic streptococcus. No toxic side-effects were noted.

REFERENCES

1 HEWITT, W. L., *J. Amer. med. Ass.*, *185* (1963) 264.
2 MCCARTHY, C. G. AND FINLAND, M., *New Engl. J. Med.*, *263* (1960) 315.
3 MCCARTHY, C. G., WALLMARK, G. AND FINLAND, M., *Amer. J. med. Sci.*, *241* (1961) 143.
4 BOND, JILLIAN M., LIGHTBOWN, J. W., BARBER, MARY AND WATERWORTH, PAMELA M., *Brit. med. J.*, *II* (1963) 956.
5 *J. Amer. med. Assoc.*, *175* (1961) 607 (Editorial).
6 WILLIAMSON, G. M., MORRISON, J. K. AND STEVENS, K. J., *Lancet*, *i* (1961) 847.
7 CHENG-CHUN LEE AND ANDERSON, R. C., *Antimicrobial Agents and Chemotherapy*, (1961) 555.
8 VOLLUM, R. L. AND JUEL-JENSEN, B. E., *Brit. med. J.*, *II* (1960) 994.
9 HALKIN, C. R., PEVNEY, D. AND ARKUS, F., *Arch. Paed.*, (1961) 57.
10 BEHRENS, O. K., CORSE, J., EDWARDS, J. P., GARRISON, L., JONES, R. G., SOPER, Q. F., VAN ABEELE, R. F. AND WHITEHEAD, C. W., *J. biol. Chem.*, *175* (1948) 793.
11 BRUNNER, R., *Öst. Chem. Ztg.*, *54* (1953) 138.
12 BOWERBANK, A. G., *Brit. med. J.*, *II* (1955) 1028.
13 GARROD, L. P., *Brit. med. J.*, *II* (1960) 527.
14 HEATLEY, N. G., *Antibiot. Med.*, *2* (1956) 33.
15 BUNN, P. A., *J. lab. clin. Med.*, *48* (1956) 392.
16 QUINN, E. L. AND COLVILLE, J. M., *New Engl. J. Med.*, *264* (1961) 835.
17 Royal College of Physicians, *Report of rheumatic fever committee*, 1957.
18 Editorials, *Brit. med. J.*, *I* (1958) 30; *II* (1962) 533.
19 BARBER, M. AND GARROD, L. P., *Antibiotics and Chemotherapy*, Livingstone, Edinburgh, London, 1963, p. 270.
20 COPE, S., SANDERSON, G., ST. HILL, C. H. AND CHAMBERLAIN, E. N., *Brit. med. J.*, *I* (1960) 913.
21 HARRIS, T. N., FRIEDMAN, S., SMITH, K. A. H., CORRELL, L. L. AND FRABRIZIO, D., *Amer. J. Med.*, *32* (1962) 545.
22 MASSELL, B. F. AND MILLER, J. M., *New Engl. med. J.*, *254* (1956) 159.
23 RUDUSKY, B. M., *J. Amer. med. Assoc.*, *185* (1963) 1004.
24 KNUDSEN, E. T. AND ROLINSON, G. N., *Brit. med. J.*, *II* (1959) 1105.
25 GOUREVITCH, A., HUNT, G. A., LUTTINGER, G. C. AND LEIN, J., *Proc. Soc. exp. Biol.*, *(N.Y.)*, *107* (1961) 455.
26 KUNIN, C. M., *Proc. Soc. exp. Biol. (N.Y.)*, *107* (1961) 337.
27 JACKSON, G. P., RUBENS, MARY AND KENNEDY, R. P., *Antimicrobial Agents and Chemotherapy*, (1961) 697.
28 KENNEDY, R. P., PERKINS, J. C. AND JACKSON, G. G., *Antimicrobial Agents and Chemotherapy*, (1962) 506.
29 GOUREVITCH, A., HUNT, G. A. AND LEIN, J., *Antibiot. Ann.*, 1959–60 (1960) 111.
30 MCCARTHY, C. G. AND FINLAND, M., *New Engl. J. Med.*, *241* (1960) 145.
31 WALLMARK, G. AND FINLAND, M., *Proc. Soc. exp. Biol. (N.Y.)*, *106* (1961) 78.
32 ENGLISH, A. R. AND MCBRIDE, T. J., *Antimicrobial Agents and Chemotherapy*, 1961, 636.

[33] CRONK, G. A., NAUMAN, R., ALBRIGHT, H. AND WHEATLEY, W. B., *Antibiot. Ann.*, 1959–60 (1960) 135.
[34] WILLIAMSON, G. M., MORRISON, J. K., AND STEVENS, K. J., *Lancet*, i (1951) 850.
[35] JACKSON, L. AND RAO, K. K., *Lancet*, i (1961) 850.
[36] NAGLEY, M., *Lancet*, i (1961) 851.
[37] ROLLO, I. M., SOMERS, G. F. AND BURLEY, D. M., *Brit. med. J.*, I (1962) 76.
[38] CARTER, M. J. AND BRUMFITT, W., *Brit. med. J.*, I (1962) 80.

Chapter 5

ACID-STABLE PENICILLINS. II

THE ISOXAZOLES; NAFCILLIN; QUINACILLIN; MISCELLANEOUS PENICILLINS

ISOXAZOLE PENICILLINS

Microbiological work with methicillin and other derivatives of 2,6-dimethoxy-benzoic acid had shown that several types of sterically hindered penicillins could be produced which resisted inactivation by β-lactamase[1]. Some of these compounds, like methicillin, shared the disadvantage of being unstable in acid and therefore unsuitable for oral administration. It was known, however, that the introduction of electron-attracting substituents into the α-position of the side-chain of benzyl penicillin produced compounds which, like the α-phenoxy penicillins, were stable in acid[2]. One class of derivatives was found to combine high activity against gram-positive cocci with stability to acid and penicillinase: this class is the 3,5-disubstituted 4-isoxazolyl penicillins[3] with the general structure (I):

(I)

$$
\begin{array}{c}
\text{R—C} \quad \text{C—CONH· CH} \quad \text{CH} \quad \overset{S}{\diagdown} \text{C—(CH}_3)_2 \\
\text{N} \quad \text{C—R'} \quad \text{C} \quad \text{N} \quad \text{CH—COOH} \\
\diagdown\text{O}\diagup \quad \text{O}\diagup
\end{array}
$$

The first compound thus prepared (II) was the 5-methyl derivative now known as oxacillin (R = C_6H_5, (R' = CH_3) wich was more active than its isomer (R = CH_3, R' = C_6H_5); several other derivatives were then examined, the most active being those with chlorine atoms in the side chain (III, IV) prepared as the sodium salts which were freely soluble in cold water.

(II) R = C_6H_5 R' = CH_3
3-phenyl-5-methyl-4-isoxazolyl penicillin (oxacillin)

(III) R = Cl   R' = CH_3
3-o-chlorophenyl-5-methyl-4-isoxazolyl penicillin (cloxacillin)

(IV)   R = Cl   R' = CH₃
3-*p*-chlorophenyl-5-methyl-4-isoxazolyl penicillin (BRL 1577)

These compounds are sufficiently acid stable for oral administration and their intrinsic activity against most pyogenic gram-positive cocci, including *Staph. aureus*, is higher than that of methicillin. They are also stable in the presence of staphylococcal β-lactamase, though less so than methicillin or quinacillin (p. 43). They can therefore be used in the oral treatment of staphylococcal infections and can be administered parenterally if higher blood and tissue levels are required. About 30% of a given dose is excreted unchanged in the urine but metabolites are also formed, probably in the liver, and excreted (see p. 124) fairly rapidly in the urine. Each derivative is protein-bound in the plasma to a higher extent than methicillin. Recent work has shown that the nature of the side chain, particularly the presence of one or more chlorine atoms, heightens activity against *Streptococcus pyogenes* as well as against staphylococci, and this may influence their usefulness clinically. At the time of writing, only two isoxazole derivatives have been approved for general issue, oxacillin and cloxacillin.

*6-(5-methyl-3-phenyl-4-isoxazolyl carboxamido)-penicillanic acid
(oxacillin, the sodium salt)*

This derivative was synthesised by the Beecham group in England and by the Bristol group in America, and produced commercially by the latter[4] after clinical trial in Syracuse, N.Y. by Bunn and Amberg[5]. These workers showed that, given orally, it was effective in infections of moderate severity due to penicillinase-forming staphylococci. This finding was soon confirmed by other workers[6-8], though it was also noted that it did not always give inhibitory serum concentrations and that its activity in this respect might be improved by further modification of the molecule (see p. 40). Its therapeutic effects too were not always reliable. Thus Huang and her colleagues[9] found that oxacillin, given orally or parenterally, was less effective than methicillin in eradicating *Staph. aureus* from the respiratory tract of children with cystic fibrosis, despite the fact that all the organisms in their series were more sensitive to oxacillin.

In common with other isoxazoles, oxacillin is rapidly absorbed, reaching peak concentration in the plasma in 0.5–1 h and declining, usually to negligible levels, in 3–6 h. There is no build-up in the serum after high doses (4 g daily) or repeated administration[10] but high plasma levels can readily be produced by giving probenecid. It diffuses, similarly to other penicillins, into milk, liquor amnii and other body fluids, but does not accede to the CSF unless given intramuscularly in large doses. It can apparently be given to pregnant and nursing mothers without injury to themselves or their infants.

Oxacillin circulating in plasma is 60–70% protein bound; even if the total protein level is lower, as in lymph, it is still nearly 50% bound[11]. This certainly interferes with its antibacterial efficacy *in vitro* but the nature of the binding, which is of the same proportion as penicillin V and phenethicillin, awaits further study. The plasma level necessary for effective therapy is probably of the order of 2–3 μg/ml and this is not always attained by oral dosage. For severe infections, parenteral use is recommended[12, 13].

Oxacillin is excreted in the urine incompletely, at a slower rate than penicillin G and methicillin. Metabolites may be formed (see p. 124). No definite toxic effects have been observed, though some investigators have noted an elevation in serum transaminase during therapy[12] which might indicate some disturbance in hepatic function.

6-(5-methyl-3-orthochlorophenyl-4-isoxazolyl carboxamido)-penicillanic acid
(cloxacillin, the sodium salt)

This isoxazole derivative of 6-APA was selected by British workers[14] as being superior to other isoxazoles. The difference is marginal and indeed the only molecular difference between oxacillin and cloxacillin is the possession by the latter of one chlorine atom in the 3-position on the benzene ring. This appears to confer slightly higher antibacterial activity, however, against staphylococci, together with better absorption, and may therefore be an asset clinically. Preliminary results suggest that this is so[15, 16]. In all other respects, cloxacillin behaves similarly to oxacillin (see above).

The first clinical trial on cloxacillin was performed by workers in 6 large hospitals, who selected for treatment patients with a variety of severe infections due to penicillinase-forming staphylococci. The results[14] in 92 patients showed that 73 were cured or much improved; failure or uncertainty of the result of treatment in the others was usually due to complicating illnesses, but two deep-seated lesions (osteomyelitis and pulmonary abscess) resisted therapy. Most of the patients received oral therapy (20–40 mg/kg/day) but it was considered essential in the most severe cases to start therapy by the intramuscular route. The drug was well-tolerated by either route; tests for renal, hepatic and haemopoietic toxicity were negative.

Since then, the clinical efficacy of cloxacillin has been confirmed by other workers[16-18] including Bunn and Kirby, who had already had extensive experience with oxacillin. If, as seems likely, cloxacillin is superior to oxacillin, there would appear to be little justification for the manufacture of both drugs.

Staphylococci are usually eliminated rapidly by cloxacillin but occassionally they persist in inaccessible sites even when the lesion itself responds to therapy, and nasal carriage is, of course, scarcely affected. As with oxacillin, staphylococci tend to persist in patients with chronic pulmonary infection (*e.g.* cystic fibrosis) and, valuable as they are in therapy, the isoxazole penicillins cannot always be relied upon to eradicate organisms from these situations. Despite their persistence and exposure to the drug, re-isolated strains of *Staph. aureus* do not acquire drug-resistance, though *Staph. albus* can readily do so.

Patients receiving cloxacillin excrete about 30% of the dose unchanged in the urine; one or more active metabolites, unidentified as yet, are also formed and excreted in comparable amounts[14-19]. The drug is also well tolerated intraventricularly, intrathecally and in infected cavities.

NAPHTHALENE AND QUINOLINE PENICILLINS

6-(2-ethoxy-1-naphthamido)-penicillanic acid
(nafcillin, the sodium salt)

This substance has a naphthalene side chain:

It was produced, along with the 2-methoxy homologue, in the Wyeth Research Laboratories, Radnor, Pa.[20], in 1961. Both naphthalene derivatives showed higher bactericidal activity *in vitro* against pyogenic cocci than methicillin. In mice infected with penicillinase-forming staphylococci, these derivatives were at least as active and, in those infected with *Str. pyogenes*

References p. 45

and *Pneumococcus*, appreciably more active than methicillin[21]. Given intramuscularly in doses of 1 g, nafcillin produced in the sera of volunteers and patients concentrations which inhibited penicillinase-forming staphylococci in titres of 1:4 or more (up to 1:128) at 1 and 2 h[22] in 87% of subjects; peak blood levels were at least four times the minimal inhibitory concentration in all the subjects. When given orally however in the same dosage (1 g), the serum levels were inadequate, even at the peak, and often not detectable. Absorption from the gut is in fact incomplete and irregular[23] so that, even when probenecid is given concomitantly, there is little or no increase in the blood level[22]. Antibacterial activity is reduced four-fold in the presence of 50% serum.

There is little detailed evidence as yet concerning the pharmacology and toxicity of nafcillin. Smith and White[24] found that 3 g daily was well tolerated orally or 2 g intramuscularly; when nasal carriers, treated intramuscularly, were usually cleared of infection—though many clinical workers would deem intramuscular therapy an unjustifiable and usually ineffective way of treating nasal carriers. The only immediate toxic effect noted was the occurrence of skin rashes in 5% of the patients. The drug is protein bound in plasma but there is no information about its distribution and metabolism. Klein and Finland[23] were able to recover only 30% of an injected dose from the urine of healthy young subjects. According to Viek[25], single doses of 1.5 g intramuscularly give consistent therapeutic concentrations in synovial fluid; nafcillin has therefore been recommended for the treatment of arthritis and osteomyelitis and, according to one report[26], is effective even when given orally (3 g daily) in patients with chronic osteomyelitis. In view of the variability of absorption reported by others workers, this finding requires confirmation.

Apart from skin rashes, there are no reports of toxicity but, with a naphthalene side-chain, the possibility of delayed toxicity cannot be excluded. The position of the drug, clinically, is uncertain at the time of writing. If certain reports [27] are confirmed, it may be comparable to the isoxazole penicillins in treating staphylococcal infections, with the advantage of higher activity if *Pneumococcus* is the infecting organism.

3-carboxy-2-quinoxalinyl penicillin (disodium salt, quinacillin)

This derivative of 6-APA is the most active of a series of quinoline and quinoxaline anhydrides prepared by the research department of the Boots Drug Company at Nottingham. The side chain is unusual:

N   CO—NH—CH———CH S C—(CH₃)₂
N   COONa   CO———N———CH—COONa

The disodium salt is stable at 100° and freely soluble in water. The presence of an electron-attracting group situated β to the amide carbonyl group in the side-chain confers a high degree of acid stability, as in ampicillin, and the quinoxaline structure causes an unusual alteration in antibacterial activity which is enhanced as the pH falls.

Quinacillin is perhaps the most selective of the penicillins in that it shows much higher activity against *Staph. aureus* than against any other pyogenic cocci (Table II). Penicillinase-forming strains are inhibited equally with those that are sensitive to penicillin G in concentrations of 0.2–0.6 μg/ml at pH 7.0, *i.e.* more active than methicillin, less active than the isoxazoles. Its action is bactericidal and it is highly resistant to staphylococcal penicillinase as well as to other sources of this enzyme. This resistance is more obvious at low than at high substrate concentrations, for quinacillin has a low affinity

TABLE II

ORDER OF BACTERICIDAL CONCENTRATIONS (μg/ml) OF THE PENICILLINS AGAINST COMMON PATHOGENS

Penicillin	Staph. aureus			Streptococcus				Gram-negative cocci		Gram-negative bacilli			
	Non-peni-cilli-nase	Peni-cilli-nase	Methi-cillin-resist.	Group A	Group D	Viri-dans	Pneu-mon.	Gono-cocci	Menin-goc.	Esch. coli	Proteus mirab.	S. typhi	Haemo-philus
nzyl (G)	**0.02**			**0.01**	5	0.1	**0.01**	0.01	**0.01**	> 10	10	**4**	2
npicillin	**0.05**			**0.01**	2	0.1	**0.01**	0.01	**0.01**	5	5	2	0.5
enoxy-(V)	0.1			0.1	> 5	1	0.1	0.5	0.5	> 20	> 20	> 10	5
enethicillin	0.2			0.2	> 10	1	0.2	0.5	1	> 50	> 50	> 20	> 5
opicillin	0.3			0.5	> 10	2	0.2		1				> 5
acillin	0.2	0.4	> 5	0.2	> 10	0.4	**0.1**		1				> 5
oxacillin	0.1	0.3	> 5	0.2	> 10	0.2	**0.4**		1	> 50	> 50	> 50	> 5
cloxacillin	0.1	0.3	> 5	0.1	> 10	0.2	**0.3**						> 5
fcillin	0.1	0.2	> 5	0.1			**0.1**	**0.1**					
ethicillin	2.5	2.5	> 20	1	> 10	4	**2**		1	> 50	> 50	> 50	> 5
enbenicillin	0.2	0.5	> 5	0.2		2	**0.2**						> 5
inacillin	**0.5**	**0.5**	> 10	2	> 10	5	**2**		> 1				>'5

here all strains of a species are sensitive, the concentration is shown in heavy type.

References p. 45

for the enzyme and is therefore inactivated very slowly at low concentrations[29]. It is also a poor inducer of the enzyme.

These properties suggest that quinacillin should be of use therapeutically in the treatment of staphylococcal infections, especially since it is not highly protein bound and shows activity when given to mice infected experimentally. However, despite its acid stability, it is poorly absorbed and has to be given parenterally. It is well tolerated by this route and shows no direct toxicity in animals or, in limited clinical trials at present in progress, in man.

A number of other alkoxynaphthoic and alkoxyquinoline carboxylic acids have also been synthesised[30]. 1,3-dimethoxy-2-naphthoic acid and 6,8-dimethoxyquinoline-7-carboxylic acid are the exact analogues of 2,6-dimethoxybenzoic acid, the side-chain of methicillin. These and other similar compounds are sterically hindered and resist inactivation by β-lactamase, in varying degree. The essential similarity of the naphthalene and quinoline nuclei, in this respect, confirms the view that insusceptibility towards this enzyme depends mainly upon the steric configuration of the side-chain. Some of these compounds show antibacterial activity but the antibacterial spectra tend to be narrow.

OTHER ACID-STABLE PENICILLINS

Acid stability in a penicillin is greatly influenced by the chemical nature of the side-chain. The best known acid stable penicillins belong to the α-aryloxyalkyl penicillin series[31] but, in all of these, acid stability is achieved at the expense of width of antibacterial spectrum. Doyle et al.[32] therefore prepared a series of α-substituted benzyl penicillins in an attempt to find an acid-stable penicillin with a wider spectrum of activity. They found that the presence of electron-attracting substituents in the α-position of the side-chain hindered degradation to penicillic acid; among other compounds, α-chloro- and α-aminobenzyl penicillin were more stable to acid than penicillins G and V, and the α-amino substituent also showed a widening of activity against gram-negative bacilli. This finding led to the preparation for therapeutic use of the more active D (−) isomer, ampicillin (Chapter 6). It was also found that 4-isoxazolyl penicillins, disubstituted in the 3- and 5-positions, combined acid stability with stability toward penicillinase, though their antibacterial spectra remained narrow.

REFERENCES

1 DOYLE, F. P., NAYLER, J. H. C., WADDINGTON, H. R. J., HANSON, J. C. AND THOMAS, G. R., *J. chem. Soc.*, (1963) 497.
2 DOYLE, F. P., NAYLER, J. H. C., SMITH, H. AND STOVE, E. R., *Nature, 191* (1961) 1091.
3 DOYLE, F. P., LONG, A. A. W., NAYLER, J. H. C. AND STOVE, E. R., *Nature, 192* (1961) 1183.
4 *Abstracts of papers presented at a Conference on Prostaphlin, Oct. 11, 1961, New York, N.Y.*
5 BUNN, P. A. AND AMBERG, J., *N.Y. St. J. Med., 61* (1961) 4158.
6 BRANCH, A., RODGER, K. C., TONNING, H. P., LEE, R. W. AND POWER, E. E., *Can. med. Ass. J., 86* (1962) 97.
7 LEDUC, A. AND FONTAINE, J., *Can. med. Ass. J., 86* (1962) 101.
8 KIRBY, W. M. M., ROSENFELD, LONA, S. AND BRODIE, JEAN, *J. Amer. Med. Ass., 181* (1962) 739.
9 HUANG, NANCY, LIBREUJAK, KATE AND HIGH, B. B., *Antimicrobial Agents and Chemotherapy*, (1962) 393.
10 PRIGOT, A., FROIX, CLEO J. AND RUBIN, E., *Antimicrobial Agents and Chemotherapy*, (1962) 402.
11 VERWEY, W. F. AND WILLIAMS, H. R., *Antimicrobial Agents and Chemotherapy*, (1962) 484.
12 *Medical Letter, 4* (1962) 29 (American edition).
13 BRAYTON, R. G. AND LOURIA, D. B., *Antimicrobial Agents and Chemotherapy*, (1962) 411.
14 STEWART, G. T. (Ed.), Report from six hospitals, *Lancet, ii* (1962) 634.
15 KNUDSEN, E. T., BROWN, D. M. AND ROLINSON, G. N., *Lancet, ii* (1962) 632.
16 KNOX, R., MACLAREN, D. M., SMITH, J. T., TRAFFORD, J. A. P. AND BARNES, R. D. S., *Brit. med. J., II* (1962) 831.
17 BUNN, P. A. AND MILICICH, SUZANNE, *Antimicrobial Agents and Chemotherapy*, (1963) 220.
18 SIDELL, S., BULGER, R. B., BRODIE, J. L. AND KIRBY, W. M. M., *Clin. Pharmacol. Ther., 5* (1964) 26.
19 ROLINSON, G. N. AND BATCHELOR, F. R., *Antimicrobial Agents and Chemotherapy*, (1962) 654.
20 ROSENMAN, S. B. AND WARREN, G. H., *Antimicrobial Agents and Chemotherapy*, (1961) 611.
21 YURCHENCO, J. A., HOPPER, MARGARET W. AND WARREN, G. H., *Antimicrobial Agents and Chemotherapy*, (1961) 620.
22 WHITEHOUSE, A. C., MORGAN, J. G., SCHUMACHER, JANET AND HAMBURGER, M., *Antimicrobial Agents and Chemotherapy*, (1962) 384.
23 KLEIN, J. O. AND FINLAND, M., *Amer. J. med. Sci., 264* (1963) 10.
24 SMITH, J. AND WHITE, A., *Antimicrobial Agents and Chemotherapy*, (1962) 354.
25 VIEK, P., *Antimicrobial Agents and Chemotherapy*, (1962) 379.
26 SMITH, L. G., *Antimicrobial Agents and Chemotherapy*, (1963) 311.
27 MARTIN, C. N., KUSHNICK, T. H., NUCCIO, P. A., GRAY, D. A., BERNSTEIN, I. AND WEBB, N. C., *Antimicrobial Agents and Chemotherapy*, (1963) 290.
28 RICHARDS, H. C., HOUSELY, J. R. AND SPOONER, D. F., *Nature, 199* (1963) 354.
29 NOVICK, R. P., *Biochem. J., 83* (1962) 229.
30 BRAIN, E. G., DOYLE, F. P., MEHTA, M. C., MILLER, D., NAYLER, J. H. C. AND STOVE, E. R., *J. chem. Soc.*, (1963) 491.
31 PERRON, Y. G., MINOR, W. F., HOLDREGE, C. T., GOTTSTEIN, W. J., GODFREY, J. C., CROST, L. B., BABEL, R. B. AND CHENEY, L. C., *J. Amer. chem. Soc., 82* (1960) 3934.
32 DOYLE, F. P., NAYLER, J. H. C., SMITH, H. AND STOVE, E. R., *Nature, 191* (1961) 1091.

Chapter 6

ACID-STABLE PENICILLINS. III
AMPICILLIN

The drug now known as ampicillin first came to the attention of the author in impure form during the period when methicillin was receiving its early trials. The light-brown powder was acid-stable and remarkably non-toxic, even when injected intravenously in animals. It was more active *in vitro* against coliforms, *Proteus* and *Haemophilus* than penicillin G and nearly as active against pyogenic cocci. The activity was however curiously and, at that time, inexplicably variable: some coliforms were rapidly killed by 2–5 μg/ml; others, apparently identical, resisted 100 μg/ml, while penicillinase-forming strains were completely resistant. In human subjects, oral absorption was usually good and well-tolerated. The compound was therefore given to two patients with refractory coliform infections of the renal tract. Both responded rapidly and, *pro tem.*, without relapse. Further tests *in vitro* showed that the mixture had a wider antibacterial range than other penicillins and that, allowing for impurity, it has the appearance of being more active than tetracyclines and chloramphenicol. In other ways, however, compound 1060 was a most dubious and unpopular substance; it was an impure mixture of two epimers; its activity was variable; it was susceptible to penicillinase; separation of the epimers was extremely difficult and costly; the evidence for therapeutic activity was slender, and yet, with a compound so impure, further clinical use would be ambiguous and unjustifiable. After a meeting at Brockham Park on October 27th, however, Farquharson decided to prepare the D(−) epimer, whatever the cost, in a quantity sufficient for further trial. This epimer, 6-D(−) α-aminophenylacetamidopenicillanic acid (BRL 1341) was used, 90% pure, for clinical trial early in 1961. After the publication of the first clinical results[1] in the autumn of 1961, this epimer was marketed and received the official name Ampicillin.

The formula of ampicillin illustrates an important point in the structure-activity properties of derivatives of 6-APA:

$C_{16}H_{19}N_3O_4S$

Mol. wt. 349

The presence of a reactive basic group (NH_2) confers or heightens activity against gram-negative bacilli (see p. 106) at pH 7.0, the free acid is sparingly water-soluble at room temperature. Solubility increases at higher pH but stability decreases. At pH 5–7, the drug is stable in solution for some hours at 37°. Ampicillin can now be prepared in a high (99%) state of purity, with a melting point of 202°. A 1% solution in water has a pH of about 4. The sodium salt is stable, more soluble, and is now used for parenteral therapy.

MICROBIOLOGY

The D(−) isomer is slightly more active than the L(+) against most organisms, but both are susceptible to hydrolysis by β-lactamase from staphylococci, coliforms and other organisms as well as to amidase from coliforms (p. 145). This limits the antibacterial spectrum to organisms which do not form these inactivating enzymes. With this limitation, ampicillin inhibits pathogenic cocci and bacilli over a wider range than any other derivative of 6-APA (Table II)[1,2]. It is nearly as active as penicillin G upon pyogenic cocci and its effect is partly or completely bactericidal.

Staphylococcus aureus. All non-penicillinase-forming strains are sensitive to 0.05–0.1 μg/ml. *Staph. albus* is similarly inhibited, 50–90% of cells being killed in 4 h.

Streptococci. All strains belonging to group A are uniformly inhibited at 0.01–0.05 μg/ml. Streptococci of other groups are also inhibited but sometimes only at higher concentrations, especially some strains of group D, *Str. viridans* and ungroupable non-haemolytic streptococci. Few strains however can resist the bactericidal effect of ampicillin at 5.0 μg/ml and a much lower concentration usually suffices. It is therefore more consistently active against streptococci than any other antibacterial drug. This property is of importance in the treatment of refractory streptococcal infections, including bacterial endocarditis (see p. 61). Pneumococci, meningococci and gonococci are also uniformly sensitive to ampicillin in slightly higher concentrations than penicillin G.

Gram-negative bacilli. In general terms, sensitive strains can be found

References p. 63/64

among many genera of the *Enterobacteriaceae* including *Escherichia coli*, paracolon bacilli and *Salmonella*. The behaviour of *Proteus* is very variable, though some strains are highly sensitive. The *Klebsiella aerogenes* group is usually resistant and *Pseudomonas* entirely so. *Haemophilus* is, usually, highly sensitive (Table II).

Escherichia coli. The behaviour of this organism depends partly upon the production of the inactivating enzymes β-lactamase and amidase. About 40% of strains from human sources form neither enzyme and the majority of these strains are sensitive in concentrations of 1–10 μg/ml, sometimes 50 μg/ml (Table III). Strains forming amidase, which may account for 50% in some situations, are moderately resistant (50–200 μg/ml). Strains forming β-lactamase are in a minority (12%) but are highly resistant (500 μg/ml or more). The action of the drug is bactericidal, even upon cells from relatively resistant strains, but never completely so. The biodynamics of ampicillin against organisms which form inactivating enzymes are complicated: a small inoculum may be suppressed before enough enzyme is produced to inactivate the drug, especially since, unlike staphylococcal penicillinase, the coliform enzymes are not readily inducible; also, at sub-inhibitory concentrations, involution forms are produced which do not divide but otherwise resist the action of the drug. Hence inoculum-size, phase of growth, genetic stability and other factors all contribute to the final result, and drug-resistance can develop quickly with exposure[1,2]. In these circumstances, coliforms and other organisms showing similar behaviour must be tested for overall sensitivity in large inocula and a bactericidal effect should be demonstrable; otherwise ampicillin is unlikely to be effective therapeutically. In their action on *E. coli*, ampicillin and penicillin G differ in degree rather than in quality. Comparable activity against *E. coli* and some other gram-negative bacilli is possessed by *p*-aminobenzyl penicillin and D-4-amino-*p*-carboxybutyl penicillin.

TABLE III

SENSITIVITY OF 134 UNSELECTED STRAINS OF *E. coli* TO AMPICILLIN AND PENICILLIN G

Inhibitory concentration (μg/ml)		Number of strains	Number of strains producing	
Ampicillin	Penicillin G		Amidase	β-lactamase
1–100	20–200	83	0	0
50–200	>500	36	36	0
>500	>500	15	—	15

Klebsiella-aerogenes group. These organisms are usually resistant to 100 μg/ml or more, often due to the production of β-lactamase which, emanating from this source, has a powerful and rapid extracellular effect. Occasionally strains are found which are inhibited by 20–50 μg/ml, but the bactericidal effect is weak.

Proteus. Some of these organisms form amidase or β-lactamase and are thereby resistant. In general, strains sensitive to 10 μg/ml are found often among *Proteus mirabilis*[3], occasionally in *Proteus vulgaris*, rarely in *Proteus rettgeri* and never in *Proteus morgani*. Even with sensitive organisms, the bactericidal effect is incomplete, involution forms and "persisters" are easily found, and drug-resistance develops quickly on passage.

Salmonella. Most strains are inhibited by 1–5 μg/ml and a strong bactericidal effect is usually obtained. No inactivating enzymes are formed by these organisms[*]. Drug-resistance does not develop readily, though it can be induced by continuous passage *in vitro*.

Shigella. Many strains, especially of *Shigella flexneri*, are inhibited by 1–5 μg/ml, but *Shigella sonnei* may be resistant to 10 μg/ml.

Pseudomonas, including *Ps. pyocyanea*, is resistant with or without the production of inactivating enzymes. A partial inhibitory effect is occasionally observed when freshly isolated strains are tested against 50–100 μg/ml. —insufficient to be of any therapeutic importance but anomalous in a penicillin, for *Pseudomonas* can usually metabolise this type of molecule.

Haemophilus. Most strains are highly sensitive to ampicillin which is often completely bactericidal at 0.5 μg/ml or less, and probably more active against this organism than any other drug.

Other organisms (Table II). Various other pathogens, including *Clostridia* and *Pasteurella*, are inhibited by ampicillin.

COMPARISON WITH OTHER ANTIBIOTICS

In view of its width of antibacterial action, ampicillin has to be compared with chloramphenicol and the tetracyclines[4], the only other major antibiotics in this category. The main difference (Table IV) is the higher intrinsic

[*] *S. Typhi-murium* (phage 1a) may be resistant to ampicillin and may form an inactivating enzyme. This resistance can be transferred in mixed cultures to *E. coli*. and thence to sensitive strains of *S. typhi-murium* (see ANDERSON, E.S. AND DATTA, NAOMI, *Lancet, i* (1965) 407).

TABLE IV

COMPARISON OF AMPICILLIN, TETRACYCLINE AND CHLORAMPHENICOL *in vitro*
(See also Rolinson and Stevens[2], Stewart *et al.*[1], Auhagen *et al.*[43])

Organism	Bacteriostatic concentration ($\mu g/ml$) and bactericidal effect (+ or −) of		
	Ampicillin	Tetracycline	Chloramphenicol
Streptococcus group A	0.01++	0.5± to 20.0−*	1.0±
Streptococcus group D	1−5+	5 to 10−*	2 to 10−*
Pneumococcus	0.01++	0.5 to 10.0±	1.0±
E. coli	1 to 5+ (20 to 500)*	5− (20 to 100)*	5− (20 to 100)*
K. aerogenes	100 to 500−	10 to 100−	5 to 50−
Salmonella typhi	0.5+	5−	2−
Salmonella typhimurium	2 to 5+	20−	5−
Proteus mirabilis	1 to 500+or−	10 to 100−	10 to 100−
Proteus morgani	>100−	10 to 100−	10 to 100−
Clostridium welchii	1 to 5+	5 to 20−	5 to 10−
Haemophilus	0.01 to 5++	1 to 5±	0.5 to 2±
Ps. pyocyanea	>100−	10 to 100−	5 to 100−

* Many strains resistant.

activity and bactericidal effect of ampicillin against sensitive organisms, especially pyogenic cocci and *Haemophilus. Pseudomonas* and the *K. aerogenes* group are more likely to be sensitive to chloramphenicol or tetracyclines, while the behaviour of *E. coli* and *Proteus* is variable. In general, it may be said that, if an organism is inhibited at comparable concentrations by all three, ampicillin is likely to have the stronger action *in vitro*. Barnett *et al.*[5] found that of *E. coli* and *Proteus* species which were resistant to tetracycline and chloramphenicol as well as to streptomycin, kanamycin and colistin, 53–88% were sensitive to less than 5 $\mu g/ml$ ampicillin, which would indicate a priority for ampicillin in the treatment of resistant infections. Tested elsewhere[1,6], the drug has been less widely inhibitory and there is evidence of considerable variation, especially in hospitals, of the sensitivity of coliforms and *Proteus*. Ampicillin and tetracyclines reach higher levels than chloramphenicol in the urine.

CROSS-RESISTANCE

When organisms are resistant to ampicillin at first isolation, they are usually cross-resistant to its L(+) isomer and to other forms of penicillin, including

p-aminobenzyl penicillin. Exceptions occur among *Proteus* spp., some strains being sensitive to penicillin G and p-aminobenzyl penicillin.

PHARMACOLOGY

Being acid-stable, ampicillin can be given by mouth, and is well tolerated and well absorbed. Peak concentrations in adults occur 1–3 h after a dose, slightly earlier in children, depending upon the state of fulness of the stomach[1,3,7,8]. Doses of 250 mg in adults give peak levels of 1–3 µg/ml which would be inhibitory to the more sensitive organisms but do not produce effective concentrations in all tissues against less sensitive organisms. If 500 mg is given, 5 µg/ml or more may be detected in the plasma, sometimes 10–12 µg/ml, which is usually adequate (Table V). Dosage should be flexible, however, within the range 20–100 mg/kg/day according to the severity of infection and response. The distribution of ampicillin in the body is similar to that of penicillin G.

Urinary excretion occurs rapidly, though not so rapidly as with penicillin G and methicillin. About 30% is excreted[7] in the first 6 h and up to 30% during the next 18 h. If dosage is given 6-hourly, a high concentration, often 1000–6000 µg/ml, is maintained in the urine[1]. When dosage ceases, the drug can be detected in the urine for the next 24 h but not thereafter if renal function is normal. The drug recovered from the urine is unaltered; metabolites, if present, are in trace amounts only. The mechanism of excretion is partly glomerular filtration, partly tubular secretion. Probenecid promotes some retention by partial blockage of tubular secretion[9]. Ampicillin is also excreted, in lesser quantity, in the bile in experimental animals and in man[10,11]. Even when large doses are given to rats, the liver copes with this elimination

TABLE V

SERUM CONCENTRATIONS OF AMPICILLIN IN ADULTS

Dose (mg)	Route	Serum or plasma concentration (µg/ml)					
		0.25 h	0.5 h	1 h	2 h	4 h	6 h
250	Oral	—	trace–3	0.3–5	3–5	0.5–1	0.1–0.3
500	Oral	—	trace–3	0.3–5	5–10*	0.5–2	0.2–0.5
1000	Oral	—	1–5	2–7	5–12*	1–3	0.2–1
250	I.M.	30	21			2	
500	I.M.	40	32			3	

* Concentrations of 20–30 µg/ml can be obtained with continuous dosage at this level. In some subjects, peak concentrations occur at about 3 h.

References p. 63/64

without signs of toxicity. The excretion product is, as in the urine, unchanged drug, much of which is immediately re-absorbed in the jejunum (Fig. 5). This process of excretion–reabsorption–re-excretion continues[11], with the result that a high concentration, bactericidal to many pathogens, is maintained in the biliary tract for some hours. Reabsorption is not quantitative

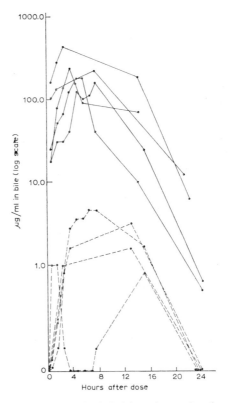

Fig. 5. Excretion and re-excretion of D(−) 6-(α-amino-α-phenylacetamido)-penicillanic acid (ampicillin) in bile of rats given 100 mg/kg. ●————● donor rats (excretion); ● - - - - - ● recipients rats (re-excretion after absorption). (Reproduced from *Brit. J. Pharmacol.*, 17 (1961) 416, by kind permission of the Editor).

due probably to some inactivation of the drug in the gut. This process serves to maintain the plasma concentration and probably accounts also for the lag in urinary excretion; but, because of this cycle, very little active drug reaches the middle and lower levels of the gut, and little or none is present in the faeces. This may limit its efficacy in treating infections of the ileum and colon. Combined renal and biliary excretion eventually reduces the plasma concentrations to ineffective levels 4–6 h after oral doses. When the drug is given parenterally, a much higher proportion is rapidly excreted in the urine and the biliary cycle is therefore shorter, though the initial concentration in the bile is higher.

In experimental animals[9], ampicillin is evenly distributed into tissues but, except in the liver and kidney, the tissue concentrations are lower than the simultaneous plasma concentrations. When dosage ceases, elimination by the mechanisms described appears to be complete. The drug does not penetrate into the C.S.F. to any extent under normal circumstances but, in patients with acute meningitis, concentrations of 3–5 μg/ml are detectable after parenteral doses at the rate of 100 mg/kg/day (see p. 61). It also accedes in concentrations of 2–4 μg/ml to pleural and joint fluid[6].

Ampicillin undergoes protein-binding in the plasma to a limited extent— less than the other acid-stable penicillins[12] and less also than chloramphenicol or tetracyclines. Such binding is probably loose and reversible. The extent, if any, to which this interferes with antibacterial activity is uncertain.

TOXICITY

Mice, dogs, rats and rabbits tolerate large doses of ampicillin by any conventional route without signs of toxicity[9]. For instance, mice and rats are unaffected by single doses, orally or subcutaneously, of 5 g/kg. If 2 g/kg is given intravenously, tremors and convulsions occur, but the animals survive. The LD_{50} intravenous appears to be about 2.5 g/kg. There are no obvious pharmacodynamic effects when the drug is given intravenously in single doses of 80 mg/kg and the local irritant action of a subcutaneous or intramuscular injection is minimal. Prolonged administration by any route at lower levels is well tolerated.

In human subjects, a number of trials reported independently disclosed no evidence of organic toxicity[4], though various side-effects have been noticed: mild diarrhoea, associated with suppression or replacement of the natural coliform flora, moniliasis, discomfort caused by swallowing the large 250 mg tablets or capsules, and skin rashes, occurring usually after the 2nd or 3rd day of treatment. These rashes have been ascribed to hypersensitivity[13] but the evidence for this is uncertain; the rashes are usually diffuse and erythematous, and occur in subjects with negative skin tests and no other signs of allergic reaction; they do not necessarily intensify and may

References p. 63/64

even disappear if dosage continues; and they are usually seen after oral, not parenteral, administration of the drug. It cannot be denied that some such reactions may be due to hypersensitivity, but it is possible that they are also due to the bactericidal action of the drug upon the intestinal bacteria, with release of endotoxins. Some patients hitherto afebrile show mild pyrexia with or without a rash at the same stage of treatment.

Irrespectively of these transient rashes, which clearly merit further study, ampicillin is strongly cross-allergenic with other penicillins and may therefore evoke any form of allergic reaction in sensitised subjects (see p. 171).

By its nature, ampicillin is often used in severe infections (renal, cardiac, respiratory) in debilitated patients. The literature to date contains many detailed records which show that oral and parenteral administration can be continued for months, in high doses, without detriment. In cases with renal infections, renal function has been noted to improve during therapy. Haemopoietic and hepatic investigations disclose no evidence of adverse effects. The intensive treatment of endocarditis, with weeks of parenteral therapy, will in due course furnish the most exacting test of toxicity; meantime, in the writer's experience, such treatment appears to cause no harm. Ampicillin has also been given intraventricularly[1] and intrathecally[14] without local toxicity.

Like all broad-spectrum antibiotics, ampicillin invariably affects the intestinal flora; being bactericidal as well, its action in this respect is singularly complete and, within a few days of commencing oral therapy, the bacterial count of the faecal flora is greatly reduced, even to zero. This effect is governed largely by the nature of the original flora. If resistant organisms or penicillinase-producers are present, these survive preferentially, while sensitive coliforms, enterococci, bacteroides and other organisms are eliminated. If therapy continues, persistent colonisation of the gut by resistant organisms ensues and may cause functional disturbance. The oropharynx may also be colonised. If the secondary flora forms amidase or β-lactamase in the absorptive area, the drug may be exposed to inactivation by these enzymes (see p. 146).

THERAPY

Though it was clear from the start that ampicillin had potential value in a variety of infections caused by gram-positive and gram-negative bacteria, the earlier trials were concerned mainly with urinary infections. A relatively high proportion of drug-resistant organisms was observed in such cases and this led many to doubt the value of the drug. Since then, however, ampicillin has found a place in a wider range of infections.

Urinary infections (Table VI)

Acute and uncomplicated infections usually respond well. This was clearly shown in a series of 45 selected cases treated by Brumfitt[3] and his colleagues at Edgware General Hospital. Sensitive organisms are quickly eliminated

TABLE VI

URINARY INFECTIONS TREATED WITH AMPICILLIN

Reference	Type of case	Organism	Number of cases		Comments
			Treated	Cured or much improved	
1	Children with abnormal renal tracts and recurring pyelonephritis	Coliforms Proteus Streptococcus group D	8	7	Rapid elimination of organisms in all cases. 2 relapsed subsequently (re-infection)
15	Miscellaneous adults	do.	41	24	Of 17 failures, 14 had resistant organisms before treatment
3	Uncomplicated acute infections	do.	45	38	Superior to nitrofurantoin, which cured 19/34 similar cases
16	Acute and chronic cystitis and pyelonephritis	do. Staph. aureus	17	8	4 failures due to resistant organisms
22	Severe chronic infections	Coliforms Proteus	12	10	2 failures due to resistant organisms
17	Obstruction with indwelling catheter	Coliforms	16	7	9 failures due to development or acquisition of drug-resistant organisms
44	Cystitis after resection of rectum	Coliforms Proteus	17	14	Best results in E. coli infections
6	Pyelonephritis and cystitis, with or without obstruction	Coliforms Proteus Others	22	18	Drug-resistance noted
		Totals	178	126(70%)	

References p. 63/64

by the bactericidal action of the drug provided it reaches the tissues as well as the urine in adequate concentration. Urinary concentrations, which are always high, may be misleading in this respect. Much depends also on the original sensitivity of the organism: highly sensitive organisms are quickly eliminated[1], even from an abnormal renal tract, but less sensitive organisms persist[15] and quickly acquire further resistance[16]. This is especially liable to occur with *Proteus* and coliforms, and careful sensitivity tests at the outset are essential. The chance of a urinary infection being due to coliforms and *Proteus* is high, but the chance of either of these organisms being sensitive to 10 μg/ml is only 50:50. Hence ampicillin should not be used blindly in this type of infection and all re-isolated organisms should be assayed afresh in case resistance is developing. Chronic renal infections are notoriously difficult to treat, especially when there is also obstruction or anatomical abnormality. In these circumstances ampicillin is probably not less useful than other drugs, but drug resistance is prone to develop and is almost certainly the main reason for failure, since most cases show lessening or disappearance of pus in the urine during the first few days of treatment. Patients with indwelling catheters[17] and obstruction are subject also to superinfection by extraneous resistant organisms during treatment.

Subject to sensitivity tests in all cases, ampicillin is most useful in controlling acute renal infections quickly; it is less valuable in chronic infections, though it still has a place; and it is unreliable in maintenance therapy though, being well-tolerated, it is often favoured for this purpose.

There are few aspects of chemotherapy in which the importance of careful laboratory control is so easily demonstrable. The overall cure rate in the first eight studies to be published was 70%, in the short term. If these reports are studied closely, it is clear that at least 18 cases should not have received ampicillin, since the organisms were insufficiently sensitive before treatment started. With these excluded from the total of 186, the cure rate rises to 79%, nearly all the failures being due to development or acquisition of resistant organisms.

Respiratory infections

The largest published series to date is that of Millard and Batten[18], who treated 52 outpatients at the Brompton Hospital, London, for chronic bronchitis. Ampicillin (500 mg twice daily) was comparable with tetracycline at the same dose over a 3-month period. There was no significant difference between the drugs in controlling symptoms and exacerbations during the winter months, or in eliminating *Haemophilus* and other pathogens from the sputum. Ampicillin seemed to cause a greater reduction in the quantity of the sputum than tetracycline. A similar study, dealing with exacerbations of chronic bronchitis, was carried out at Hammersmith Hospital by Ayliffe and Pride[19]. In this trial, ampicillin was compared with dimethylchlortetracycline and penicillin V plus streptomycin; ampicillin was effective, but not more so than the other drugs. In an earlier pilot trial with a smaller series of cases, Grant et al.[20] reported a similar result. There is therefore general agreement that, in the management of chronic bronchitis, ampicillin is as eligible as tetracyclines, which are now widely and, on the whole, effectively used for this purpose. Both drugs produce side-effects during long-term therapy and the choice of which to use depends partly on this: in infants and children, tetracyclines must be used with caution on account of their interference with dentition and skeletal growth[21]; but, in patients with any form of penicillin-hypersensitivity or allergic diathesis, ampicillin is contra-indicated. There is undoubtedly a continuing place for both drugs in the chemoprophylaxis of respiratory infection in bronchitic and other subjects, especially in controlling exacerbations provoked by *Pneumococcus* and *Haemophilus*.

Ampicillin has also been found useful in the treatment of other forms of respiratory infection. Zylka et al.[16] in Cologne used it in a variety of infections, some of which were secondary to lesions such as bronchial carcinoma, and reported satisfactory results in 37 out of 49 cases. Several oɪ their patients showed skin rashes, thought to be allergic. Trafford et al.[15] and Lockey et al.[22] in London found ampicillin uniformly effective in eliminating *Haemophilus* in chronic infections; when bronchiectatic cavities were infected by coliforms or *Proteus* the results were much less satisfactory. Bunn et al.[6] in Syracuse, N.Y., were impressed by the efficacy of the drug in 8/8 cases of pneumococcal lobar pneumonia, though resolution was delayed or absent in 3/6 patients with gram-negative pneumonia. In respiratory infections, drug-resistance and active superinfection have been much less frequent than in urinary cases treated with ampicillin, though it is common experience that colonisation of the oropharynx with penicillinase-forming coliforms can readily occur. In infants, or in patients with bronchiectasis, such organisms can perhaps interfere with further recovery, but they seldom cause active infection and can usually be disregarded.

Acute pneumonia in newborn infants is a paediatric emergency in which ampicillin can be useful[23], especially while bacteriology is pending. This type of infection may be due to gram-negative as well as to gram-positive organisms, amenable to the width of spectrum of ampicillin though, if penicillinase-forming staphylococci are present, or thought to be present, another drug such as cloxacillin should be given as well. This combination is useful also in the long-term therapy or chemoprophylaxis of mucoviscidosis (fibro-cystic disease) where staphylococcal infection or superinfection is a grave menace. So far, ampicillin has mainly been given orally for respiratory infections but, for severe infections, there are advantages in beginning treatment with intramuscular injections to replace the large oral doses (2–3 g/day) recommended by Zylka[16] and other investigators. In minor infections (mild bronchitis, sinusitis) oral doses of 1 g/day are usually sufficient.

It has been known for years that penicillin G (and tetracyclines) have some action on viruses of the psittacosis–lymphogranuloma group[24], possibly because these organisms have mucopeptide cell walls containing muramic acid[25] which make them comparable to small gram-negative bacilli multiplying within cells. Allison and Busby had the interesting idea that ampicillin, with its wider activity, might inhibit these organisms more effectively than penicillin G and proceeded to test their hypothesis by comparing the two penicillins for their ability to inhibit the mouse pneumonitis virus, a representative member of the group. Their results[26], though unconfirmed as yet, bore out the theory convincingly, for ampicillin was at least twice as active as penicillin G in inhibiting the development of lethal lesions in mice. If further experimentation supports these findings, there might be a place for ampicillin in the chemoprophylaxis or treatment of disease in man caused by these viruses. The applicability of the finding to other viruses is doubtful, for the psittacosis–lymphogranuloma group is different, structurally and biochemically, from most others.

Alimentary infections

The bactericidal action of ampicillin on *Salmonella* led to the belief that it would be useful in treating cases and carriers of this type of infection. In cases, it has to be compared with chloramphenicol[27], which is undoubtedly effective in systemic infection by *Salmonella typhi*, *Salmonella paratyphi B* and other *Salmonella*. For the clearance of carriers, no single drug or combination of drugs is reliable, though many are in constant use for the purpose. In assessing any drug against *Salmonella* in patients, these two aspects of the infection have to be differentiated; it must be remembered also that many *Salmonella* cause only a localised, self-limiting enteritis with a spontaneous clearance-rate which is probably as high as that produced by any antibacterial drug. Nevertheless, typhoid and paratyphoid fever are hurdles in therapy which still have to be cleared, and a critical assessment of ampicillin in this field is important.

Isolated successes have been reported by Maddock[28], Trafford et al.[15], Patel[29], Kennedy et al.[30]. The first controlled trial reported was that by Murdoch and his colleagues[31] in a major outbreak of infection by one strain of S. paratyphi B (phage type Taunton) in Edinburgh. These workers compared ampicillin in relatively large doses (6 g/day in adults, 200 mg/kg/day in children) with standard doses of chloramphenicol (2 g or 75 mg/kg) in a random, cross-over trial in which treatment with the other drug was substituted after 10 days in patients not responding to the first drug, which was otherwise continued for 14 days. 60 patients, of all ages, were treated initially with chloramphenicol, 80 similar cases with ampicillin, the organism being present in the stools or blood cultures, or both, in all cases. Maximum blood levels with chloramphenicol were about 8 μg/ml as against 32 μg/ml with ampicillin; since ampicillin is intrinsically more active against the organism, this concentration should have given it a distinct advantage in eradicating systemic infection. In the trial, however, the patients' temperatures fell to normal more rapidly with chloramphenicol, though subjective improvement seemed to occur at about the same rate. The bacteriological relapse rate was slightly lower in cases receiving ampicillin. No drug resistance against either antibiotic was found in re-isolated organisms, nor was there any evidence of toxicity. From this it can be concluded that ampicillin in high doses is a useful alternative to chloramphenicol but not necessarily superior.

In weighing the merits and demerits of these two drugs, the physician must also be influenced by their comparative toxicities. Ampicillin is devoid of direct toxicity but it can cause skin reactions and may be dangerous in allergic subjects. Chloramphenicol is usually well tolerated in a first course but, in second or subsequent courses, carries an increasing risk of haemopoietic damage, which may be fatal. With ampicillin the dose can be increased or given with safety parenterally; with chloramphenicol this would be hazardous. If infection is localised in the biliary tract, as in some carriers, ampicillin is preferable.

In infections due to other Salmonella, ampicillin is equally eligible for use, though unproved, when infection is systemic. Early attempts to disinfect intestinal carriers of Salmonella, among other pathogens, were disappointing[1, 32, 33], but recent work by Christie[34], of Liverpool who treated eight chronic carriers of S. typhi with large doses for three months, holds promise. His dosage was:

References p. 63/64

1st week:

BRL 1060 (isomers of ampicillin)	500 mg i.m. 6-hourly
Ampicillin	1 g orally 6-hourly
Probenecid	1 g orally twice daily

2nd–12th weeks:

| Ampicillin | 1 g orally three times a day |
| Probenecid | 1 g orally twice daily |

Christie used BRL 1060 (see p. 46) because, at the time of his trial, an injectable preparation of ampicillin was not available and he was convinced from the failure of previous efforts that high dosage was essential. Of his eight carriers, all of whom had been identified bacteriologically years beforehand and kept under surveillance for five months before the trial, seven became negative and remained so for a year following treatment. In six, a hundred consecutive stools were negative; in one, 34 out of 34 specimens were negative; in the eighth case, 44 out of 44 stools were negative in the three months after treatment but thereafter *S. typhi* was again excreted in the stool and was also isolated from duodenal bile.

Though less conclusive than Christie's results, reports by Troy[35] and Geddes[36] show that ampicillin is capable of curing carriers of *S. typhi* and *S. paratyphi B*, while that of Coles[37] shows that carriers of *Shigella sonnei* and *E. coli* serotypes can also be cleared of infection. The secret probably lies in the intensity and duration of treatment. In chronic carriers the organism is presumably locked in inaccessible sites perhaps intracellularly, and a high reservoir of bactericidal drug must therefore be maintained in the plasma and tissues to kill any organisms which are released. Ampicillin has an advantage over all other drugs attacking gram-negative bacilli, for it is bactericidal at concentrations of 0.5–5.0 μg/ml and non-toxic in levels, easily attainable, which are far above this. If it can clear carriers of *S. typhi* and *S. paratyphi*, it will be the only drug to do so, out of many tested. *Salmonella* are, in general, inhibited by 5 μg/ml or less but there are some strains, especially of *Salmonella typhimurium*, which resist 20 μg/ml. When the organism has been re-isolated from treated cases or carriers, drug-resistance has not been observed but this minority of relatively-resistant strains has not been encountered in clinical trials as yet.

If these results are confirmed in larger trials and in infections with other *Salmonella*, there may be a stronger case for using ampicillin instead of, or subsequently to, chloramphenicol during the acute stage of infection, especially during epidemics, to lower the number of convalescent carriers. Murdoch's results[31] show a trend in this direction. There is no evidence of any advantage in giving the two drugs simultaneously; indeed, the bacterio-static action of chloramphenicol might conceivably interfere with the bactericidal effect of ampicillin.

Meningitis

Ampicillin is highly active against all the organisms usually responsible for primary pyogenic meningitis, and may usefully be given while the bacteriological diagnosis is pending. Wehrle and his colleagues give it intravenously in doses of 100–150 mg/kg/day during this period, and often continue this regime with benefit[38] (see p. 178). In meningitis due to atypical streptococci and *E. coli*, ampicillin may be the drug of choice. It can be given intrathecally and intraventricularly with impunity[1,14].

Septicaemia and endocarditis

Bunn[6] and his colleagues report good results in 11/12 cases with positive blood cultures, often with immediate sterilisation. The writer has had similar experience in 5 patients with pneumococcal, streptococcal, staphylococcal and coliform bacteriaemias. One of Bunn's patients had endocarditis due to *Str. viridans*, which responded quickly. The writer has collaborated with colleagues in treating 3 cases of endocarditis, 2 being due to streptococci of group D and one to an ungroupable streptococcus which had failed to respond to saturation therapy with penicillin G. In each of these cases, ampicillin was given intramuscularly (100 mg/kg/day) for 4–6 weeks, then orally for 3 months; in one case, cessation of treatment during this time precipitated a relapse. Endocarditis due to group D streptococci is notoriously difficult to treat and, for some years, combined therapy with penicillin G and streptomycin has been favoured[39]. Ampicillin is perhaps the only single drug with consistently high activity against these and related streptococci and is certainly eligible for therapy in such infections, provided it is given parenterally. Quinn *et al.*[40] found the bacteriostatic effect of ampicillin against enterococci no greater than that of penicillin G but, if the bactericidal effects are compared, ampicillin is usually more active against these and related streptococci.

References p. 63/64

Other infections

In the biliary tract, ampicillin attains higher concentrations than any other antibiotic at present in use[41]. It can therefore be used, as Zylka[16] and Bunn[6] have shown, with good clinical results, in biliary infections and as a prelude to or accompaniment of biliary surgery. Successful results have been reported also in wound infections, peritonitis and pelvic sepsis[1,6,15,42,43]. In any of these situations, more than one organism may be present, and sensitivity may vary; the possible presence of penicillinase-forming coliforms and of drug-resistance should also be borne in mind.

GENERAL CONCLUSIONS

At the time of writing, less than three years have elapsed since the publication of the first clinical report upon ampicillin. During that time, published work from Europe and America has established its value as a broad-spectrum antibiotic with a range of therapeutic activity comparable to that of tetracyclines or chloramphenicol. If hypersensitivity reactions are excluded, its toxicity is much lower and its intrinsic bactericidal activity higher than these drugs. Its main use might lie in the chemoprophylaxis and therapy of respiratory infections, but it is also highly eligible for many urinary infections, meningitis, septicaemia, endocarditis, peritonitis, biliary infections and pelvic sepsis. In some situations, especially in the urinary tract, drug resistance may develop during therapy if the infecting organism is a coliform or *Proteus*. Despite its width of antibacterial activity, ampicillin fails to inhibit certain gram-negative bacilli and is higly susceptible to the action of penicillinase from staphylococci or other organisms. Careful sensitivity tests, with large inocula of the organism under test, must therefore be performed in all cases and repeated if the organism is re-isolated.

Ampicillin is less active *in vivo* against *Salmonella* than its behaviour *in vitro* would suggest. The reasons for this are complex, but it can be used, in large doses, as an alternative to chloramphenicol in systemic infections due to these organisms. Preliminary, but carefully evaluated, trials in chronic carriers of *S. typhi* indicate that large doses, preferably given parenterally as well as orally, can cure the carrier state; this may apply also to other *Salmonella* if care is taken to exclude a minority of resistant strains.

REFERENCES

[1] STEWART, G. T., COLES, H. M. T., NIXON, H. H. AND HOLT, R. J., *Brit. med. J.*, *II* (1961) 200.
[2] ROLINSON, G. N. AND STEVENS, SHIRLEY, *Brit. med. J.*, *II* (1961) 191.
[3] BRUMFITT, W., PERCIVAL, A. AND CARTER, M. J., *Lancet*, *i* (1962) 130.
[4] STEWART, G. T., *Pharmakotherapia*, *1* (1963) 197.
[5] BARNETT, J. A., SANFORD, J. P., FERGUSON, R. A. AND PERRY, NANCY E., *Antimicrobial Agents and Chemotherapy*, (1962) 350.
[6] BUNN, P., O'BRIEN, J. BENTLEY, D. AND HAYMAN, H., *Antimicrobial Agents and Chemotherapy*, (1962) 323.
[7] KNUDSEN, E. T., ROLINSON, G. N. AND STEVENS, SHIRLEY, *Brit. med. J.*, *II* (1961) 198.
[8] KIENITZ, V. M., *Arzneimittel-Forsch.*, *12* (1962) 802.
[9] ACRED, P., BROWN, D. M., TURNER, D. H. AND WILSON, M. J., *Brit. J. Pharmacol.*, *18* (1962) 356.
[10] BROWN, D. M. AND ACRED, P., *Brit. med. J.*, *II* (1961) 197.
[11] STEWART, G. T. AND HARRISON, PATRICIA M., *Brit. J. Pharmacol.*, *17* (1961) 414.
[12] SCHOLTON, W. AND SCHMID, J., *Arzneimittel-Forsch.*, *12* (1962) 741.
[13] *Brit. med. J.*, Editorial, (1964) *I*.
[14] SPITTLE, C. R. AND PHILLIPS, B. M., *Postgrad. med. J.*, *38* (1962) 168.
[15] TRAFFORD, J. A. P., MACLAREN, D. M., LILLICRAP, D. A., BARNES, R. D. AND HOUSTON, J. C., *Lancet*, *i* (1962) 987.
[16] ZYLKA, VON W., CHRISTNER, M. AND MOERS, H., *Arzneimittel-Forsch.*, *12* (1962) 803.
[17] VINNICOMBE, J., *Lancet*, *i* (1962) 1186 (corresp.).
[18] MILLARD, F. J. C. AND BATTEN, J. C., *Brit. med. J.*, *I* (1963) 644.
[19] AYLIFFE, G. A. J. AND PRIDE, N. B., *Brit. med. J.*, *II* (1962) 1641.
[20] GRANT, I. W. B., DOUGLAS, A. C. AND MURRAY, W. D., *Brit. med. J.*, *II* (1962) 483.
[21] *Lancet*, Editorial, *2* (1963) 283.
[22] LOCKEY, EUNICE, EATON, B. R. AND COMPSTON, N., *Brit. J. clin. Pract.*, *16* (1962) 13.
[23] BEARGIE, R. A. AND RILEY, H. D., *Antimicrobial Agents and Chemotherapy*, (1963) 331.
[24] HAMRE, D. AND RAKE, G., *J. infect. Dis.*, *81* (1947) 175.
[25] ALLISON, A. C. AND PERKINS, H. R., *Nature*, *188* (1960) 796.
[26] ALLISON, A. C. AND BUSBY, D. *Brit. med. J.*, *II* (1962) 834.
[27] HUCKSTEP, R. L., *Typhoid fever and other Salmonella infections*, Livingstone, Edinburgh, 1962.
[28] MADDOCK, C. R.. *Lancet*, *i* (1962) 918.
[29] PATEL, K. M., *Lancet*, *i* (1963) 1387.
[30] KENNEDY, W. P. U., WALLACE, A. T. AND MURDOCH, J. McC., *Brit. med. J.*, *II* (1963) 962.
[31] SLEET, R. A., SANGSTER, G. AND MURDOCH, J. McC., *Brit. med. J.*, *I* (1964) 148.
[32] ROSS, S., LOVRIEN, E. W., ZAREMBA, E. A., BOURGEOIS, L. AND PING, J. R.,*J. Amer. med. Assoc.*, *182* (1962) 238.
[33] TYNES, B. S. AND UTZ, J. P., *Ann. intern. Med.*, *57* (1962) 871.
[34] CHRISTIE, A. B., *Brit. med. J.*, *I* (1964) 1609.
[35] TROY, PATRICIA, *Brit. med. J.*, *I* (1964) 1252.
[36] GEDDES, A. M., *Postgrad. med. J.*, *40* (1964) Suppl.
[37] COLES, H. M. T., *Postgrad. med. J.*, *40* (1964) Suppl.
[38] IVLER, D. THRUPP, L. D., LEEDOM, J. M., WEHRLE, P. F. AND PORTNOY, B., *Antimicrobial Agents and Chemotherapy*, (1963) 335.
[39] CATER, J. E., CHRISTIE, R. V. AND GARROD, L. P., *Brit. med. J.*, *I* (1951) 653.

[40] QUINN, E. L., COLVILLE, J. M., BALLARD, L., JONES, D. AND DEBNAM, F., *Antimicrobial Agents and Chemotherapy*, (1962) 339.
[41] HARRISON, PATRICIA M. AND STEWART, G. T., *Brit. J. Pharmacol.*, *17* (1961) 420.
[42] HOLLOWAY, W. J., PETERS, C. D. AND SCOTT, E. G., *Antimicrobial Agents and Chemotherapy*, (1963) 314.
[43] AUHAGEN, E. VON, *et al.*, *Arzneimittel-Forsch.*, *12* (1962) 792.
[44] PENDOWER, J.E.H., *Practitioner*, *189* (1962) 65.

Chapter 7

COMPARISON OF THE ORAL PENICILLINS

If the various oral penicillins all possessed the same antibacterial properties, comparison would be simple and would be made in terms of their pharmacological efficiency. In fact, they differ considerably in antibacterial spectra and intrinsic activity, which are the primary considerations. They must therefore be grouped in terms of these considerations before comparison can be made.

(1) Broad-spectrum and high intrinsic activity: Ampicillin
Penicillinase-susceptible.

(2) Narrow-spectrum, penicillinase-resistant: Oxacillin
    Cloxacillin
    Nafcillin

(3) Intermediate spectrum, penicillinase-susceptible: Penicillin V
(the phenoxypenicillins)   Phenethicillin
    Propicillin
    Phenbenicillin

(1) No other penicillin with width of activity comparable to ampicillin has yet been described. With the exception of penicillinase-forming staphylococci, all pathogens are more sensitive to ampicillin than to any of the other oral penicillins listed. If oral penicillin therapy is contemplated, and if cost is not a deterrent, ampicillin gives the widest cover; if penicillinase-forming staphylococci are present, along with other pathogens, or are likely to be present, ampicillin should be given along with one of the drugs in group *(2)*.

(2) Of the penicillinase-resistant oral penicillins at present available, cloxacillin possesses the highest intrinsic activity against pyogenic cocci[1] and gives better, more consistent plasma levels after comparable oral doses than the others. The decision as to which should be used is not, therefore, in doubt, but it should be remembered that severe staphylococcal infections

require parenteral, not oral, administration in the first place; for this purpose, cloxacillin again appears to be preferable.

(3) Differences between the phenoxypenicillins are more difficult to evaluate. Phenoxymethyl penicillin (penicillin V) is the most active and inhibits some organisms (streptococci, pneumococci) much more effectively than the other phenoxy derivatives. Also, it should be remembered that penicillin G itself is partly absorbed when given orally in sufficient dosage[2]; this absorption has been found adequate in the past for the control of bacterial pneumonias[3] and for eliminating nasopharyngeal streptococci from children[4]. Being less active against these organisms, and narrower in range, the other phenoxypenicillins are useful only in so far as their improved absorption might permit a corresponding improvement of active and available drug-level in the plasma and tissues; this in turn is influenced by protein-binding, rate of excretion and other factors whose significance has not been fully assessed.

If absorption of these penicillins be taken as a criterion, it is now well-established that phenethicillin[5-7], propicillin[8] and phenbenicillin[9] at equal doses produce higher total concentrations in the plasma than penicillin V. Some workers have denied that these differences are important[10,11], while others claim that propicillin[8] and phenbenicillin[9] produce more effective levels than phenethicillin.

The results obtained with these substances seem to show major variations if there are minor differences in the methods of assay. Thus Bond et al.[12], diluting serum for assay in premedication serum from the same subject, found no significant difference between total antibiotic level produced by dhenethicillin and propicillin, though phenbenicillin gave higer levels, whereas Williamson et al.[13], using pooled sera in buffer as diluent, found that propicillin gave levels twice as high as phenethicillin.

The total serum or plasma concentration comprises a variable protein-bound fraction plus free drug. Protein binding occurs with all penicillins but varies greatly in degree. In the plasma, the fraction affected is the albumin, to which penicillin is bound loosely and reversibly. This binding is usually thought to interfere with antibacterial action[14] and, with the new as well as the older penicillins[15,16] the interference is more or less proportional to the extent of the binding. Binding occurs readily *in vitro* as *in vivo*, but is diminished by dilution; hence the well-known technical discrepancy whereby a serum diluted in saline of buffer gives a higher figure on bio-assay than one which is diluted in serum or albumin, or tested without dilution. Standards for comparison have to be made up and treated similarly and, unless these technical factors are carefully controlled and standardised, comparative studies of the drugs are misleading. Of the four phenoxypenicillins, phenbenicillin and propicillin are more highly protein bound than phenethicillin or penicillin V, in that order[16]. The extent to which this process interferes with absorption, excretion and release to the tissues is unknown (see p. 34). Stereoisomeric factors also play a part, as in the case of phenethicillin, whose L-isomer or D-L mixtures give more active serum concentrations than the D-isomer[17].

Estimates of total serum concentration are therefore misleading in comparisons of these drugs (Table VII). Concentration of free drug (*i.e.* not bound) can be made by dialysing the serum or plasma under negative pressure. When this is done[12], phenethicillin and penicillin V give higher levels, at equivalent dosage, than propicillin or phenbenicillin.

TABLE VII

BEHAVIOUR OF α-PHENOXYPENICILLINS AFTER A GIVEN ORAL DOSE

Total concentration in serum	Phenbenicillin > propicillin or phenethicillin > penicillin V
Protein binding	Phenbenicillin > propicillin > phenethicillin > penicillin V
Unbound fraction	Phenethicillin > penicillin V > propicillin > phenbenicillin

The effectiveness of a given level of antibiotic, free or bound, depends also upon the net bactericidal action, which varies with the antibiotic and the organism. To make allowance for this, Colville and Quinn[16] calculated the percentage efficiency of a given drug as:

$$\frac{\text{MIC in broth}}{\text{MIC in serum}} \times 100$$

Bond *et al.*[12] preferred to estimate the fold increase in MIC caused by the presence of serum, and also estimated the ratios

$$\frac{\text{Total blood level}}{\text{MIC in serum}} \quad \text{and} \quad \frac{\text{Free blood level}}{\text{MIC in broth}}$$

As a mode of study, these and similar ratios serve to express more lucidly the antimicrobial efficiency of a given drug against a given organism in a given fluid; as such, they are probably better than any other estimates at

References p. 69

present available, but it should nevertheless be borne in mind that the albumin binding of penicillin, among other drugs, is a reversible process which decreases with the loss of free drug to the tissues or excretory channels[18]. The effectiveness of unbound drug in the plasma at an arbitrary time may not wholly represent its therapeutic potential. With this reservation, the ratios of Bond *et al.* and of Colville and Quinn show fairly close agreement: penicillin V and phenethicillin are superior to phenbenicillin and to a lesser extent to propicillin against *Staph. aureus* and *Str. pyogenes* when given in equal doses.

Even if the net effective blood level is an adequate criterion of therapeutic efficacy, careful assessments such as those described above may be incomplete. Some authorities prefer to look at the "area under the curve" (*i.e.* the measurable area beneath the line joining the points forming it) as an indication of the total effective antibacterial activity of the plasma during that time[17]; others prefer to take the peak as a measurement of the quantity available for diffusion into the tissues. By these criteria, phenbenicillin and then propicillin would be judged superior to phenethicillin and penicillin V. Then again, the absolute quantities of total and free drug acceding to infected sites is undoubtedly important, and there is little data about this; protein binding, which interferes with activity *in vitro*, may serve to retain the drug in inflamed tissues or to stabilise the equilibrium between plasma and tissue. The rate of inactivation and excretion, and the presence of active metabolites (see p. 126) might also be relevant. In some infections, the maintenance of a prolonged bacteriostatic concentration might be more useful than the bactericidal effect which is so important in endocarditis or septicaemia. These factors are at present imponderable, from lack of data. The final judgment will depend upon the clinical efficacy of the drugs but, since none is entirely inactive, this will await carefully controlled trials and the passage of time. In these circumstances, it is impossible either to favour or dismiss any of these drugs, but it can be said that the advantages, if any, of the later derivatives are marginal. Penicillin V or, for that matter, large doses of penicillin G, given orally are of proven efficacy. Until more data accumulates it would seem wise to use these drugs for the infections which are known to respond and to reserve the others for cases failing to respond. In view of the variability of absorption of some penicillins, it is also advisable to estimate blood levels with some regularity whenever there is any doubt over the efficacy of a given derivative.

REFERENCES

1 KNOX, R., MACLAREN, D. M., SMITH, J. T., TRAFFORD, J. A. P. AND BARNES, R. D. S., *Brit. med. J.*, *II* (1962) 831.
2 BUNN, P. A., *J. lab. clin. Med.*, *48* (1956) 392.
3 FLIPPIN, H. F., MATTEUCCI, W. V., SCHIMMEL, N. H. AND BOGER, W. P., *J. Amer. Med. Assoc.*, *147* (1951) 918.
4 WEHRLE, P. F., FELDMAN, H. A. AND KURIDA, K., *Pediatrics*, *19* (1957) 208.
5 MORIZI, E. M. E., WHEATLEY, W. B. AND ALBRIGHT, H., *Antibiot. Ann.*, *7* (1959–60) 127.
6 PERRON, Y. G., CRAST, L. B., GOTTSTEIN, W. J., MINOR, W. F. AND CHENEY, L. C., *Antibiot. Ann.*, *7* (1959–60) 107.
7 KNUDSEN, E. T. AND ROLINSON, G. N., *Lancet, ii* (1959) 1105.
8 WILLIAMSON, G. M., MORRISON, J. K. AND STEVENS, K. J., *Lancet, i* (1961) 847.
9 ROLLO, I. M., SOMERS, G. F. AND BURLEY, D. M. *Brit. med. J.*, *I* (1962) 76.
10 McCARTHY, C. G. AND FINLAND, M., *New Engl. med. J.*, *263* (1960) 315.
11 GRIFFITH, R. S., *Antibiot. Med.*, *7* (1960) 129.
12 BOND, JILLIAN M., LIGHTBOWN, J. W., BARBER, MARY AND WATERWORTH, PAMELA M., *Brit. med. J.*, *II* (1963) 956.
13 WILLIAMSON, G. M., MORRISON, J. K. AND NAYLOR, P. G. D., *Brit. med. J.*, *II* (1963) 1588 (corresp.).
14 TOMPSETT, R., SCHULTZ, S. AND McDERMOTT, W., *J. Bact.*, *53* (1947) 581.
15 KUNIN, C. M., *Proc. Soc. exp. Biol. (N.Y.)*, *107* (1961) 337.
16 COLVILLE, J. M. AND QUINN, E. L., *Antimicrobial Agents and Chemotherapy*, (1961) 600.
17 *J. Amer. med. Assoc.*, *175* (1961) 607 (Editorial).
18 ZINNEMAN, H. H., HALL, W. H., HONG, L. AND SEAL, U.S., *Antimicrobial Agents and Chemotherapy*, (1962) 637.

Chapter 8

METHICILLIN

Steric hindrance to the attachment of enzyme to substrate may or may not be conceptually correct in the final forum of molecular biology, but it was this concept which gave birth to methicillin, the first therapeutic penicillin to withstand the action of staphylococcal penicillinase and, thereby, to inhibit resistant staphylococci. After a few preliminary experiments with hindered acids (p. 26), methicillin (BRL 1241) was produced from dimethoxybenzoic acid and 6-APA. Its antibacterial spectrum was narrow, its intrinsic activity only one-hundredth that of penicillin G; but it inhibited penicillinase-forming staphylococci in large inocula equally with non-penicillinase-forming staphylococci, and was not appreciably inactivated by the enzyme. Unlike its hindered precursors, it appeared to be devoid of any immediate toxicity to animals.

This much was ascertained at Brockham Park, but external factors then intervened. At that time, in 1959, hospital-bred infections with resistant staphylococci were becoming an uncontrollable menace (p. 179). The chief medical adviser to the Beecham companies, Dr. E. T. Knudsen, formerly of the Middlesex Hospital, was aware of the urgency of this type of infection, and organised without delay human trials in volunteers among the personnel of the Company and at Guy's Hospital Medical School. An opportunity also arose to give the drug both intramuscularly and intravenously to a patient in the Middlesex Hospital seriously ill with staphylococcal infection post-operatively following cardiac surgery. These studies, necessarily brief, confirmed the fact that the drug was non-toxic in the short-term. Clinical trials were then organised at Guy's Hospital and Queen Mary's Hospital for Children, Carshalton, where "bandit" bacteria were being studied. History repeated itself in a curious way. It will be recalled (p. 13) that one of the first cases treated informatively at Oxford with the original penicillin was a 2-month child with multiple foci of osteomyelitis; the second patient treated at Queen Mary's with methicillin was practically identical, the penicillinase-forming staphylococcus having been acquired in a maternity hospital. Sterilisation of the blood culture and clinical improvement in this infant was the first clear-cut indication of the therapeutic potency of methicillin. The clinical trial was extended and all the investigators concerned met at the Apothecaries' Hall in May 1960 to exchange information. At this meeting, plans were made for the publication of laboratory and clinical data, which appeared in the *British Medical Journal* of September 3rd and the *Lancet* of September 10th[1-9].

Methicillin was marketed also in America by the Bristol Company under a different trade name. Production and clinical trial had been impeded there by technical difficulties which were overcome after a visit by Chain and Farquharson on the occasion of the opening of Bristol's new laboratories by the Governor of New York State, Mr. Nelson Rockefeller, in October 1959. If the immediate impact of methicillin in the United States was less noticeable than in Great Britain, the resultant clinical activity was much greater and, within a few months, many more reports were available[10-13] to confirm and amplify the British publications. In all these early studies, large doses were given without evidence of toxicity, though cross-allergenicity was noted in a few patients known to be hypersensitive to penicillin G[2,4].

PROPERTIES OF METHICILLIN

Methicillin is sodium 6-(2,6-dimethoxybenzamido)-penicillanic acid monohydrate (Fig. 6). It is freely soluble in water but highly unstable to acid and must therefore be administered parenterally. In concentrations of 1–3 μg/ml it is bactericidal to the great majority of strains of *Staph. aureus* and also to

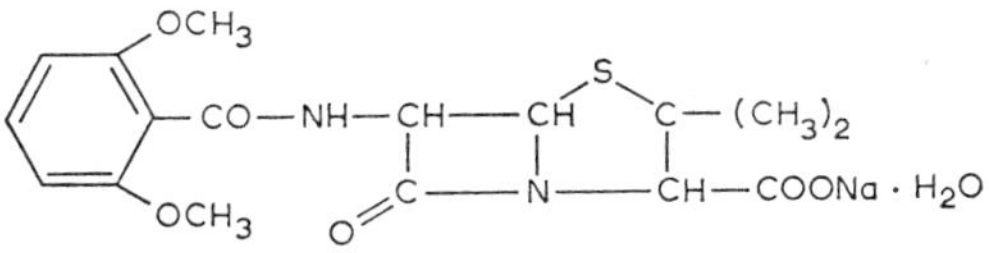

Fig. 6. Sodium 6-(2,6-dimethoxybenzamido) penicillate monohydrate.

certain other pyogenic cocci such as pneumococci and streptococci of group A which are uniformly sensitive within this dose range. Other streptococci are much less sensitive and gram-negative bacilli completely insensitive. Methicillin is therefore a narrow-spectrum substance of comparatively low activity when compared with penicillins G or V. Its action on staphylococci

References p. 79/80

is due to the fact that the molecule is insusceptible to the β-lactamase produced by these organisms[1] though not necessarily to other forms of this enzyme[4]. Despite its insusceptibility to hydrolysis, methicillin has a high affinity for staphylococcal β-lactamase and, in sub-inhibitory concentrations of about 0.5 μg/ml, is an excellent inducer of the enzyme. This kind of inducement, in the words of Knox[14] is the "frenzied formation of a futile enzyme", but it has been the means of showing that many staphylococci which form no β-lactamase when growing normally do so if an inducing substrate is added. A fuller description of the interaction between inactivating enzymes and substrate is given in Chapter 13.

It is only rarely that staphylococci are naturally resistant to methicillin. When the drug was first introduced, some 5000 strains were examined before a naturally-resistant strain was isolated[15] and this strain was distinctly abnormal, probably non-pathogenic. Since then a few resistant strains with limited invasiveness have been identified[16-18]. This subject is discussed in more detail in Chapter 13, but it can be said here that natural or drug-induced resistance to methicillin on the part of *Staph. aureus* is extremely rare and, as a clinical problem, unimportant as yet. There is evidence[19] that *Staph. albus* may behave differently in this respect, for continued therapy with methicillin may transform a sensitive into a resistant strain. This has to be borne in mind during the treatment of endocarditis and other cryptic lesions due to this organism by methicillin or other penicillins, for cross-resistance tends to be complete.

PHARMACOLOGY AND TOXICITY

Being unstable to acid, methicillin is unsuitable for oral administration. When injected intramuscularly or intravenously it is well-tolerated, though some pain may result from intramuscular injection and, to minimise this, procaine is sometimes included in the dose. Plasma concentration and tissue distribution are similar to those obtained with comparable doses of penicillin G.

As far as is known, the drug circulates in the plasma largely in the free form, with less protein-binding than penicillin G[9]. The drug also enters lymph in higher concentration than other penicillins[20]; in this fluid, as much as 94% may be in the free form. It is rapidly excreted in the urine of human subjects[5] and several animal species[21] in unchanged form, with no evidence of metabolic conversion in man[4]. This excretion, which is both glomerular and tubular[21] accounts for 75–80% of the injected dose and, if the renal tract is normal, the bulk of this is excreted within 4 h of a given injection. Of the remainder, 2–3% is excreted in the bile during the first few hours after an injection[22] and then destroyed in the gut. As with ampicillin, the ratio of bile: blood concentration is higher than that of penicillin G.

Even when very high doses are given to animals, there is no evidence of direct toxic action on the liver, kidneys or other major organs. Mice tolerate 2.5 g/kg intravenously but show occasional clonic convulsions after 3–5 g/kg. Continued dosing of 500 mg/kg to young rats causes no interference with growth. No adverse effects are seen in electrocardiographic, respiratory or blood-pressure tracings when the drug is given intravenously in doses far in excess of those used therapeutically.

Methicillin has now been given to tens of thousands of patients on a very extensive scale indeed and is almost always well tolerated. Babies have received 104 g in 76 days without toxicity[23]; adults have received 500 g or more during the long-term treatment of endocarditis and osteomyelitis[24] and many more patients have now been under surveillance for three or more years after treatment. Some cases originally treated by the writer have now been followed for five years and have shown no evidence of toxicity. There is therefore overwhelming evidence that methicillin is one of the least toxic of all antibacterial drugs. Nevertheless, a few reports from experienced workers have been published suggesting that it can very occasionally cause trouble. McElfresh and Huang[25] recorded a case of granulocytopenia in which the depressed cell count returned immediately to normal when methicillin therapy was terminated. Few other similar cases have been recorded, though the author has been informed by Maxwell Finland that three similar occurrences in America were reported to him. The batches of methicillin responsible were not available for analysis. Any interference with leucopoiesis must obviously be rare in the extreme, for leucocyte counts have regularly been done in patients receiving high doses of methicillin and usually indicate an unimpeded granulocyte response. Following the appearance of McElfresh and Huang's paper, the writer repeated the haematology in twelve patients who had received large doses of methicillin in the original trial; none of these cases showed any abnormality, nor was granulocytopenia provoked by subsequent injections of the drug. At a later date, granulocytopenia was noted in an infant under treatment for empyema; the blood picture in this case was highly abnormal, for there was also a congenital haemoglobinopathy with anaemia; these abnormalities persisted after methicillin was withdrawn and may have been already present. Hewitt et al.[26] have recorded eosinophilia,

References p. 79/80

along with renal and other abnormalities, in three patients receiving methicillin but, in all three, there was also a leucocytosis. There is therefore no evidence that methicillin has any direct action upon the marrow, but the possibility of very occasional idiosyncrasy cannot be discounted until more data is available.

There is also limited evidence of disturbance of renal function in patients receiving methicillin. Hewitt and his colleagues quote three cases each showing oliguria and haematuria accompanied by eosinophilia and fever between the 14th and 28th days of therapy. One was a case of endocarditis, the second was probably hypersensitive to penicillin, and the third was also receiving vancomycin; nevertheless, in each case renal function improved and the other signs subsided when methicillin was discontinued. Penicillin hypersensitivity can display itself in varied symptomatology, but renal manifestations are extremely uncommon[27-29] and, in two recorded cases, was accompanied by purpura, which Hewitt's cases did not show. Allen et al.[30] noted signs of renal damage and hypofunction in two patients receiving methicillin for septicaemia but the signs subsided while the drug was continued and were presumably due to the septicaemia. Grattan[31] in a careful study of one case, a child who developed haematuria on three occasions during methicillin therapy, found no evidence of permanent renal damage at autopsy but considered that the drug might have caused a transient glomerular lesion. In this case haematuria appeared on the 3rd–5th day of the second and subsequent courses of the drug and was not noted during the first course. The six cases so far recorded therefore show only two common features—signs of renal damage and insufficiency, and severe infections; the other features differ considerably from case to case.

From this data, it can be concluded that sudden signs of renal damage may appear when methicillin is being used to treat severe infections; there is no proof that it is directly nephrotoxic in itself and, indeed, this possibility would seem to be discounted by the rarity of these occurrences and by the tolerance, by various animals and man, of huge doses. It is always possible that an abnormal metabolite might be formed, but this was not studied in the six cases described and methicillin is, in fact, less likely to yield detectable metabolites than phenethicillin or the isoxazoles, which have not been associated with renal damage. Also, methicillin is well-tolerated by patients with certain renal lesions such as those caused by infection. The evidence of nephrotoxicity, such as it is, points to the glomerulus as the vulnerable site. Until more is known, methicillin should be used with care in patients with a history of glomerulonephritis; in all other patients it would seem enough if the very occasional possibility of renal damage is kept in mind, especially when repeated courses are being given.

Independently of toxicity, methicillin is locally irritant when injected into a muscle, as is penicillin G. To minimise this, local anaesthetic can be given with the injection. This can best be done[32] by first injecting 0.5 ml of 1% lignocaine, disconnecting the syringe and injecting methicillin from a second syringe 15 sec later.

THERAPY

Methicillin is specifically indicated in one condition and one condition only: staphylococcal infection where there is any possibility that the organism has been acquired by cross-infection, especially in hospital, and is consequently resistant to penicillin G. In severe infection of this type, proved or suspected, methicillin is the drug of first choice. If the organism is subsequently found to be sensitive to penicillin G, methicillin should be discontinued and penicillin G given instead. When a methicillin-treated infection comes under control, one of the isoxazole penicillins may be substituted to avoid needless prolongation of injections.

Dosage should be viewed flexibly, according to the site and severity of the infection. Abscesses, pneumonia and wound sepsis may resolve on the minimum dose schedule of 20–50 mg/kg/day (250–500 mg 6-hourly in an adult); empyema and osteomyelitis require at least 50 mg/kg/day for longer periods, two months or more in the case of osteomyelitis; in septicaemia and pyaemia the drug should be given in the range 50–100 mg/kg/day with injections 4-hourly during the first day or two; in endocarditis 5–10 g should be given daily to adults. It is usually wise, in these severe infections and in meningitis, to give the drug intravenously in the first instance. A convenient method is to dissolve the 4-hourly dose in 200 ml saline and give this by a slow intravenous drip with intermittent boosting doses of 500 mg or more through a side-arm in the needle. In meningitis, 2–20 mg should also be given into the CSF until the organisms disappear.

The threshold of bactericidal activity is abrupt, more so than with any other penicillin. The drug may kill 90% of an inoculum at 2 μg/ml but be without significant effect at 1 μg/ml. The plasma (and tissue) level should therefore be maintained at not less than 2–3 μg/ml, which is the average bactericidal concentration, for as long as possible. When severe infections are being treated, this level may be increased without hesitation until plasma levels not lower than 15 μg/ml are obtained at some stage. An intramuscular

References p. 79/80

injection of 1 g usually produces this concentration in the plasma within 0.5 h, dropping by half at 1–2 h and to the threshold level of 1–2 μg/ml after 3–4 h[4,5,10]. Excretion is delayed by giving probenecid[33,34] and higher blood levels maintained. Severe infections have been treated with 24 g/day for several weeks without detriment[35].

The original clinical trials established the fact that methicillin, like penicillin G, had a rapid detoxifying effect in patients with staphylococcal septicaemia, pneumonia, osteomyelitis and other severe lesions; local signs of inflammation also subsided rapidly and, in many but not in all instances, the infecting staphylococci were eradicated from the main site of infection. The drug appeared to be more active in these respects than erythromycin, tetracyclines or chloramphenicol; an equally rapid antibacterial effect could sometimes be obtained with vancomycin, but this drug is toxic and continued dosage difficult. The immediate success of methicillin was undoubtedly due to its visible curative power in severely-ill patients who had ceased to improve on treatment by the other drugs then available. Whether or not it retains pride of place in such cases is now less certain, even though, at the time of writing, over four hundred references to its use have been traced in international medical literature, and few of these cite any major disadvantages other than those mentioned above. Newer drugs are now available, however, including the isoxazole penicillins (p. 38) which have higher intrinsic activity and are acid-stable. There is evidence also that, in staphylococcal pneumonia and osteomyelitis, the new steroid antibiotic fucidin may show appreciable activity. Nevertheless it is important to remember that methicillin has had a longer and more exacting trial than any newer antistaphylococcal agent and that, more than any other single factor, it dealt with the resistant staphylococcus so effectively that the epidemic menace has now dwindled to manageable proportions. In 1959 the columns of the *Lancet* and of the journals of the American and British Medical Associations carried four editorial references and over forty other entries dealing specifically with hospital staphylococci; in 1963 these same editors expressed popular relief by their silence.

The *Lancet*[36] drew attention to "*Staphylococcus domesticus*" in lieu of "*Staphylococcus infirmarius*". In the *British Medical Journal*[37] the main reference was to the possibility of resistance to the new penicillins, which could reinstate the menace. Having been blooded in this race, methicillin still enjoys the status of champion and it is very important that some careful clinical and epidemiological revaluation of its contemporary prowess be made, now that new rivals are in the field. With this reservation, methicillin can still be regarded as the pre-eminent drug for the control of resistant staphylococcal infections, meriting use to the limit of dosage in such cases, and also probenecid (0.5 g four times a day) to prolong blood levels if necessary.

PROPHYLACTIC USE OF METHICILLIN

There are various theoretical reasons for restricting or even avoiding the use of methicillin prophylactically. In practice, the matter has seldom been put to the test, so that factual data is scanty. The first attempt to use methicillin in this way was a bold one. Elek and Fleming[38] investigated the effect of spraying methicillin in maternity wards to control staphylococcal cross-infection; their idea was that droplet nuclei of antibiotic would thereby enter the patients' nostrils in the same way as the organisms, and suppress colonisation. The results, assessed from repeated nasal swabs, were impressive for not only was the incidence of colonisation and infection by staphylococci reduced; a stage was even reached in a few months when the wards were virtually cleared of the organisms. Drug-resistance was not encountered during this period. In a subsequent study[19] of the effect of spraying upon the induction of resistance, the writer found that *Staph. aureus* gradually disappeared in the manner described by Elek and Fleming, but that it was often replaced by *Staph. albus* which could acquire resistance to the drug readily on exposure, *in vitro* and *in vivo*. This may be of importance clinically in surgical wards containing patients for cardiac or neural operations where infection with *Staph. albus* is a serious problem[23]. There is no doubt however about the immediate efficacy of spraying methicillin in eliminating *Staph. aureus*, even if only an individual spray is used[39,40]. The effect of spraying on nasal carriage is temporary and probably does not lessen the liability to subsequent infection[41].

Nasal carriage is a major but by no means sole source of staphylococcal infection. Goldfarb and James[42], studying the problem in thoracic surgical wards, considered that infected sputum was also a likely source. In one ward, with a record of several closures due to cross-infection, they sprayed methicillin daily throughout the ward and its main annexes for a year, and also gave methicillin by injection pre- and post-operatively to all their patients during the first six months. New patients, with infections, were admitted throughout the period. During the first few weeks of the trial, two patients acquired cross-infections, each of which responded under the (routine) therapy with methicillin. Thereafter, no cross-infections were observed and the incidence

References p. 79/80

of staphylococci in nasal swabs and sputa fell amost to zero. These workers had been assiduous in trying other drugs and procedures before they resorted to methicillin and they were convinced that "a genuine eradication of cross-infection was brought about by this procedure where other measures based on different principles failed". The principle of the spraying method is to achieve and maintain a concentration of dust-like particles of antibacterial agent in the atmosphere; when methicillin is used, the inhalation of these particles progressively eliminates staphylococci from the respiratory tract and, as a result, the feed-back of organisms into the atmosphere is stopped and cross-infection from this major source prevented. There is no doubt, from numerous other studies [43–45] of the importance of nasal reservoirs of infection and, in situations where this is a special risk, that a reversion to the Listerian practice of spraying would clearly be desirable if a satisfactory anti-bacterial agent could be found. Whether methicillin should be used in this way is still debatable. Continuous exposure of patients to the drug provides a seemingly perfect situation for the promotion of contact hypersensitivity, or for provoking reactions in subjects already sensitised, including some nurses who might well be in a state of dangerous sensitisation. Curiously enough, no such occurrences have been noted in the various studies so far conducted, but it is known that methicillin is cross-allergenic with and cross-antigenic to other penicillins and the risk therefore stands (see Chapter 14).

The absence of drug-resistance on the part of *Staph. aureus* is understand-able. Continuous exposure of this organism to therapeutic or sub-therapeutic levels does not render it resistant to methicillin or, as far as we know, to other penicillins; even *in vitro* the organism has to be passaged intensively through rising concentrations of the drug before resistance develops. Such resistance as has been encountered clinically seems to depend upon the existence, in an extreme minority of group I and III strains, of organisms with an intrinsic capacity to withstand the bactericidal action of the drug and to grow, usually abnormally, in its presence (Chapter 13). If such organ-isms were present in any one patient, survival would surely be selectively favoured by the presence of methicillin, and it is known that they can cause cross-infection[16,18]. *Staph. albus* is not usually a problem but, in surgical wards and in infants, its presence cannot be ignored, and here it is known that drug-resistance can be induced quickly by exposure to therapeutic levels of methicillin. In the light of these facts, the general use of methicillin (or any other major antibiotic) for spraying is unjustifiable but, when adequate and critical bacteriological supervision is available, spraying on a restricted scale may serve to prevent or arrest cross-infection in vulnerable situations.

In respiratory infections with staphylococci, clinical improvement is not always accompanied by simultaneous disappearance of the pathogen, irrespectively of which antibacterial drug is used. In any patient, with any type of lesion, passive nasal carriage of staphylococci may persist during and after intensive oral or parenteral dosage[4]. From the epidemiological viewpoint it is therefore important to examine sputum and nasal swabs for persisting organisms and, if cross-infection is feared or if epidemic strains are harboured, to attempt to eliminate them by aerosols or intranasal disinfectants.

REFERENCES

[1] ROLINSON, G. N., STEVENS, SHIRLEY, BATCHELOR, F. R., CAMERON-WOOD, J. AND CHAIN, E. G., Lancet, ii (1960) 564.
[2] DOUTHWAITE, A. H. AND TRAFFORD, J. A. P., Brit. med. J., II (1960) 687.
[3] KNOX, R., Brit. med. J., II (1960) 690.
[4] STEWART, G. T., HARRISON, PATRICIA M. AND HOLT, R. J., Brit. med. J., II (1960) 694.
[5] KNUDSEN, E. T. AND ROLINSON, G. N., Brit. med. J., II (1960) 700.
[6] STEWART, G. T., NIXON, H. H. AND COLES, H. M. T., Brit. med. J., II (1960) 703.
[7] THOMPSON, R. E. M., WHITBY, J. L. AND HARDING, J. W., Brit. med. J., II (1960) 706.
[8] THOMPSON, R. E. M., HARDING, J. W. AND SIMON, R. D., Brit. med. J., II (1960) 708.
[9] BROWN D. M. AND ACRED, P., Lancet, ii (1960) 568.
[10] BUNN, P. (Ed.), Symposium on dimethoxyphenyl penicillin, State University of New York, Syracuse, 1960.
[11] RUTENBURG, A. M., GREENBERG, H. L. AND SCHWEINBURG, F. B., New Engl. med. J., 263 (1960) 1174.
[12] BULLOCK, W. E., JR., Antimicrobial Agents and Chemotherapy, (1961) 770.
[13] HUANG, NANCY N. AND HIGH, R. H., Antimicrobial Agents and Chemotherapy, (1961) 787.
[14] KNOX, R., Guy's Hosp. Rep., 110 (1961) 134.
[15] JEVONS, M. PATRICIA, Brit. med. J., I (1961) 124.
[16] STEWART, G. T. AND HOLT, R. J., Brit. med. J., I (1963) 308.
[17] HARDING, J. W., J. clin. Path., 16 (1963) 268.
[18] BOROWSKI, J., KAMICUSKA, KAROLINA AND RUTECKA, IRENA, Brti. med. J., I (1964) 983.
[19] STEWART, G. T., Brit. med. J., I (1961) 863.
[20] VERWEY, W. F. AND WILLIAMS, H. R., Antimicrobial Agents and Chemotherapy, (1962) 484.
[21] ACRED, P., BROWN, D. M., TURNER, D. H. AND WRIGHT, D., Brit. J. Pharmacol., 71 (1961) 70.
[22] HARRISON, PATRICIA M., WHITE, JEAN A. AND STEWART, G. T., Brit. J. Pharmacol., 15 (1960) 571.
[23] CALLAGHAN, R. P., COHEN, S. J. AND STEWART, G. T., Brit. med. J., I (1961) 860.
[24] HEWITT, W. L., J. Amer. med. Assoc., 185 (1963) 264.
[25] McELFRESH, A. E. AND HUANG, NANCY, New Engl. J. Med., 266 (1962) 246.
[26] HEWITT, W. L., FINEGOLD, S. M. AND MOUZOU, O. T., Antimicrobial Agents and Chemotherapy, (1961) 765.
[27] SPRING, M., J. Amer. med. Assoc., 147 (1951) 1139.
[28] UNGAR, A. M. AND NEMUTH, H. I., J. Amer. med. Assoc., 167 (1958) 1237.

[29] WARWICK, W. J., *Minnesota Med.*, *43* (1960) 484.
[30] ALLEN, J. D., ROBERTS, C., EVANS, J. AND KIRBY, W. M. M., *New Engl. J. Med.*, *266* (1962) 111.
[31] GRATTAN, W. A., *J. Pediat.*, *64* (1964) 285.
[32] DOUTHWAITE, A. H., TRAFFORD, J. A. P., McGILL, D. A. F. AND EVANS, I. E., *Brit. med. J.*, *II* (1961) 6.
[33] STEVENSON, F. H. AND HARRISON, K. J., *Brit. med. J.*, *II* (1960) 1596.
[34] HENDERSON, W. R., CARLETON, JUDITH AND HAMBURGER, M., *Amer. J. med. Sci.*, *243* (1962) 489.
[35] BRANCH, A., RODGER, K. C., LEE, R. W. AND POWER, E. E., *Can. med. Assoc. J.*, *83* (1960) 991.
[36] *Lancet*, *ii* (1963) 235.
[37] *Brit. med. J.*, *I* (1963) 280.
[38] ELEK, S. D. AND FLEMING, P. C., *Lancet*, *ii* (1960) 569.
[39] STRATFORD, B., RUBBO, S. D., CHRISTIE, R. AND DIXSON, S., *Lancet*, *ii* (1960) 1225.
[40] BARBER, MARY AND WARREN, S., *Lancet ii*, (1962) 374.
[41] ULSTRUP, J. C. AND ØDEGAARD, A., *Lancet*, *ii* (1961) 1227.
[42] GOLDFARB, SUSAN AND JAMES, G. C. W., *Brit. med. J.*, *I* (1963) 305.
[43] WILLIAMS, R. E. O., NOBLE, W. C., JEVONS, M. PATRICIA, LIDWELL, O. M., SHOOTER, R. A., WHITE, R. G., THOM, B. T. AND TAYLOR, G. W., *Brit. med. J.*, *II* (1962) 275.
[44] ROUNTREE, P. M., HARRINGTON, M., LOEWENTHAL, J. AND GYE, R., *Lancet*, *ii* (1960) 1.
[45] LOEWENTHAL, J., *Brit. med. J.*, *I* (1962) 1437.

Chapter 9

THE MODE OF ACTION OF PENICILLINS. I

MORPHOLOGICAL AND BIOCHEMICAL APPROACHES

Now that penicillins can be designed to attack resistant as well as sensitive organisms while yet retaining their non-toxicity to mammalian cells, the study of their mode of action offers insight into fundamental aspects of bacterial physiology as well as to the rational therapy of infection. This study is now evolving, as it should, into an interdisciplinary alloy of biochemistry, biophysics and microscopy, but microbiologists from simpler schools of thought, like the writer, can still find solace in the thought that, twenty years ago, direct observations on bacteria led even then to conclusions which are now being confirmed in more sophisticated terms.

EARLY OBSERVATIONS

Fleming saw that the effect of penicillin upon sensitive pyogenic cocci was essentially bacteriolytic, though he noted that lysis was often preceded by a period of preliminary growth. The Oxford workers also noted that, in liquid cultures, the lytic effect occurred after a preliminary increase in turbidity. Gardner[1] found that this could be due to swelling of individual cells rather than to growth, though growth could occur before death of the cells[2,3] at optimal concentrations. The Oxford team also found[4] that penicillin did not lessen the oxygen uptake of suspensions of staphylococci and had little direct effect on cells which, in suspension, were in the resting state. Thus was born the important idea that penicillin acted mainly upon dividing cells. Confirmation that the effect was bactericidal came from several laboratories[5-10]. Chain, with the late E.S. Duthie[11], then showed that, at low concentrations (0.04–0.1 unit per ml), penicillin caused an increase in oxygen consumption by cultures of staphylococci for about 1.5 h and then a fall to zero; at higher concentrations (1 unit per ml) there was no initial rise before the fall but, within this range, penicillin was inhibiting the respiration of dividing cells prior to their dissolution. Hobby and her colleagues, and Lee *et al.*[3], claimed that the bacterial count rose and then fell, but Chain and Duthie did not find this. It became apparent, from the work of Todd[12] and others, that the result depended upon the organism used and concentration of penicillin added. Some organisms, like pneumococci and *Str. pyogenes*, were rapidly killed by low concentrations but other organisms persisted, with abnormal morphology; bacteriostatic as well as bacteriolytic effects were being observed and, with some organisms, the result depended upon the inoculum added as well as upon the concentration of drug. Meanwhile, the Oxford workers had discovered penicillinase in certain coliforms, and this appeared to explain the insusceptibility of some gram-negative bacilli.

MORPHOLOGICAL CHANGES

The swelling of staphylococci noted by Gardner was also observed in other organisms exposed to penicillin. This occurred *in vivo* as well as *in vitro*—in those days it was readily observed in urethral smears from military patients with gonorrhoea—and was clearly a rapid consequence of contact between sensitive bacterial cells and penicillin. In sensitive cells, abnormalities of size and shape frequently occurred before death but the bactericidal action was not always complete. Bigger[8] gave the name "Persisters" to staphylococci which withstood lysis amid predominantly-sensitive populations. It was noted also that some gram-negative bacilli, such as *Proteus*, hitherto regarded as resistant, could be inhibited by relatively low concentrations of penicillin[13] and that "persisters", insensitive to these low concentrations, were thereby selectively preserved. Despite their high resistance to the drug, these persisting organisms showed variations in colonial and other properties which appeared to be due to their contact with penicillin. Involution forms appeared also in intestinal bacilli exposed to sub-inhibitory concentrations[14]. It appeared therefore that penicillin had an effect upon a wider range of bacterial cells than was originally thought, but the nature of this effect was far from clear to most observers. The idea that penicillin acted optimally upon dividing cells was established but this action was somethimes bactericidal, sometimes bacteriostatic, sometimes incomplete, depending upon concentration of drug, age of culture, type of organism and other unknown factors.

Amid this uncertainty, a speculative observation by Duguid[15] stands out in precognition of later findings. Studying the elongated and swollen bacillary forms produced by penicillin, this worker suggested that growth without division could be due to the failure to form outer supporting cell-wall material and that the locus of action might be the cell wall itself. Some other interesting findings, still unexplained, were recorded at that time by Eriksen[16] also using the technique of direct agar microscopy[17] of colonies growing from single cells exposed to penicillin. He found that staphylococci did not as a rule undergo lysis without preceding growth; in weak concentrations, growth was characterised by large, shadow-like cells which died but did not disappear whereas, at higher concentrations (1 unit per ml) this swelling did not occur and lysis was incomplete or absent. In contrast, pneumococci underwent complete lysis, with disappearance, at any concentration, though swelling occurred only at low concentrations. This provided direct evidence of the selective toxicity of penicillin to dividing staphylococci but suggested that other organisms were affected differently. In a subsequent study[18], Eriksen considered that the action of penicillin upon various representative organisms (gram-positive cocci and bacilli, gram-negative bacilli) differed according to whether high or low concentrations were used: high concentrations caused lysis without preceding growth or swellings, whereas low concentrations caused lysis only when preceded by primary growth or swelling or both. Meanwhile, other studies[19] indicated that the morphological effects of penicillin were most marked upon gram-negative bacilli which were much less susceptible to lysis. This linked up with Duguid's contention[15] that penicillin had a specific action upon all bacterial cells. Viewed in this light, sensitivity was a relative term, definable by the levels attainable in plasma and tissues by conventional dosage. Since penicillin was non-toxic, organisms hitherto deemed resistant might be brought within its ambit of sensitivity by employing higher doses. It will be recalled that in those critical early years, penicillin was in short supply and that dosage was based largely upon the schedules devised with painstaking and cheeseparing accuracy for pyogenic coccal infections in Oxford; had penicillin G been given originally in doses of 1–2 g/day (equivalent to 1.7–3.3 mega units), like tetracyclines and chloramphenicol, it might have been classified as a broad-spectrum antibiotic. In the present day, when marginal improvements are offered as advances in therapy, it is useful to apply a little simple arithmetic. Even so, in clinical as well as microbiological terms, the main action of penicillin was directed against the pyogenic cocci; gram-negative bacilli were collectively much less vulnerable. Studies on mode of action habitually differentiated the sensitive gram-positive coccus from the resistant gram-negative bacillus.

References p. 95/97

BIOCHEMICAL POINTERS

In all its essentials, this fundamental difference in sensitivity had been revealed by microbiological work. The first chemical clue to the nature of the difference came in the observation by Gale and Taylor[20] that penicillin prevented the transportation of glutamic acid into the cell substances of staphylococci from an external medium containing peptides and glucose. This effect was not obtained with a gram-negative coliform bacillus similarly treated. These findings, pursued by Gale and his colleagues during the next few years, led to further knowledge about the interrelationships between nucleic acid and protein synthesis in bacterial cells; but it proved to be mainly a reflection, not an explanation, of the mode of action of penicillin in high concentrations. Meanwhile, two other promising biochemical openings were being probed.

In 1949, Park and Johnson[21] found that labile phosphate accumulated in cells of *Staph. aureus* grown in the presence of penicillin in very low concentrations. The accumulated phosphate, which was acid-soluble, was quickly identified[22] as a complex of three compounds, each containing uracil, two phosphate groups, pentose and an unknown sugar; two of the compounds contained amino acids. It seemed that synthesis of these compounds, which was accelerated by glucose, occurred only during the period of growth and swelling (noted earlier by Gardner[1]), 30–45 min after exposure to penicillin, while the cells were still viable. During this period the effect of penicillin at 0.5 μg/ml was greater than that at 0.1 μg/ml.

Uptake of penicillin by bacteria

At about the same time, Maas and the same Johnson[23] in America, and Rowley, Cooper and their colleagues in England[24], found that penicillin was to some extent bound by staphylococci. It will be recalled that Gale[20] had already shown that penicillin prevented the transport of glutamic acid across the cell wall of staphylococci and, further, that organisms trained to grow in the absence of given amino acids became resistant without exposure to penicillin[25]. This suggested that the action of the drug on staphylococci was an interference with uptake of amino acids. Rowley and Cooper reasoned that if an organism required energy to transport preformed amino acids from the external medium into the cell, it would be sensitive to penicillin which appeared to inhibit this process. Microbiological assay disclosed no uptake of penicillin by cells but radioactive studies, using penicillin labelled with ^{35}S, showed minute but specific binding with a component present in resting staphylococci in cell suspensions. During early growth, binding increased, presumably because more of the binding component became available to the penicillin. Maas and Johnson used biological as well as radioactive methods of assay and found that binding of penicillin was firm; unlike Rowley and Cooper, they found no correlation between this minute binding and the sensitivity of the organism to penicillin. Nevertheless, the facts that pre-treatment with crystalline penicillin prevented the uptake of labelled penicillin, and that uptake increased with growth, led Rowley and his colleagues to the conclusion that binding was a specific feature of the action of penicillin and that organisms with a high affinity for binding were more highly sensitive.

By 1950, therefore, and with remarkably little theorising, a number of salient points about the action of penicillin had been noted: the initial swelling of susceptible cocci; the vulnerability of dividing cells; the elongation without division in relatively resistant gram-negative bacilli; the interference with amino acid transport into sensitive cells and the accumulation therein of an unfamiliar labile phosphate complex; and the irreversible uptake of penicillin by sensitive cells during early growth. At this stage, none of the investigators responsible for these observations, except Duguid, had postulated the cell wall as the site of action but it was clear that the lesion caused by penicillin was highly specific.

Relevant structures in the bacterial cell

To understand the next steps, it is helpful to review briefly the structure of a bacterial cell, particularly its subdivision into an inner, cytoplasmic cell body enclosed by a limiting osmotically-active membrane and an outer, relatively rigid cell wall. Substances essential for metabolism, growth and multiplication tend to be concentrated within the cell body; these include nucleic acids and their precursors, proteins, amino acids, phosphates and phosphate esters together with a battery of enzymes. Most of these substances can be released by surface-active agents[26] with death of the cell but preservation of some enzyme activity. In lysozyme-sensitive bacteria, the cell wall can be dissolved completely by this enzyme; in other organisms the walls can be more or less completely removed by suspending them in liquid made hypertonic by the addition of non-penetrating crystalloids such as sucrose or sodium chloride. The naked cell body or protoplast is thereby liberated but remains intact only if the osmotic pressure of the surrounding medium is of the same order as that within the cytoplasm. Given this equilibrium, protoplasts survive and grow slowly, containing within their cytoplasm the main components, including the enzymes, of the intact cell[27]. The limiting cytoplasmic membrane, being impermeable to many substances, acts as an osmotic barrier. If the osmotic pressure of the surrounding medium falls, the high pressure retained within the protoplasts causes it to burst. Under normal conditions, this is prevented by the strong cell wall; hence any damage to the cell wall, or any imperfection in its synthesis during growth and division, may lead to lysis.

Changes in cellular metabolites

Between 1950 and 1952, Park proceeded to identify his three phosphate complexes which accumulated in penicillin-treated staphylococci. Using aqueous phenol and partition chromatography[28], he found that all three compounds consisted of uridine, labile and stable phosphates, and a potential reducing substance; all three had the same basic unit of structure, namely uridine 5-phosphate attached to an amino sugar by an acetyl-like bond[29]. When differentiated further[30], each of the three compounds appeared to be unique in that they possessed an N-acetylamino sugar and amino acids in combination with a nucleotide. These compounds ("Park nucleotides") were found to be present in trace quantities (< 0.1 μg/g wet weight) in normal staphylococci, increasing fifty-fold in cells treated with penicillin. Compound 1 is the basic unit; compound 2 contains an L-alanine residue; compound 3 contains a peptide chain of L-lysine, D-glutamic acid and three D/L-alanine residues (Fig. 7).

It was apparent from this work that nucleotides of unusual structure, present in traces in normal staphylococci, began to accumulate when the cells were exposed to penicillin. Accumulation within the cells was maximal when the cells were just growing, at the threshold of the bacteriostatic concentration (< 0.1 μg/ml), and occurred during the first 30–45 minutes, along with swelling and growth of the cells. When the cells were no longer viable, accumulation ceased. This corresponded to the time, known from other work, at which lysis began to occur.

The Park nucleotides were perhaps the strongest clue to the mode of action of penicillin in 1952, but they were not the only clue. Gale's work indicated that there was also interruption of amino acid uptake: it had been shown that, in the presence of a complete mixture of amino acids and glucose, staphylococci formed combined glutamate instead of free glutamic acid, and peptides appeared in the external medium[31]. If purines and pyrimidines were added to this mixture, nucleic acid synthesis was increased[32]. No nucleic acid was formed in the absence of amino acids but, if amino acids were present in optimal proportions for protein synthesis, nucleic acid syn-

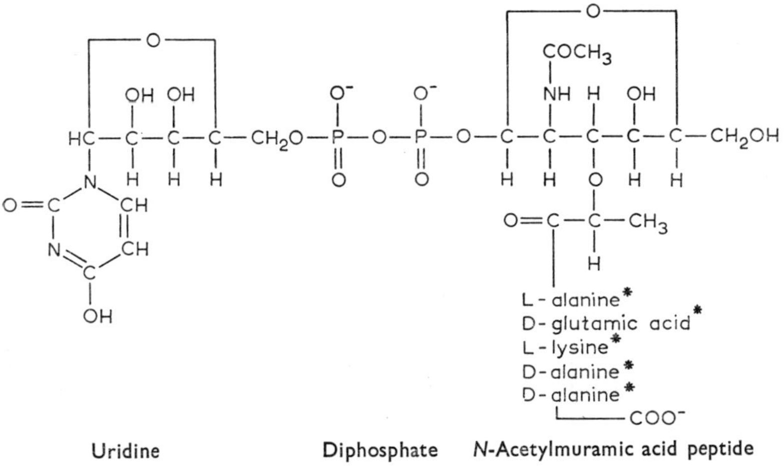

Fig. 7. Structure of uridine disulphate N-acetylmuramic acid (Park nucleotide).
* The amino sugar and these amino acids are present in normal staphylococcal cell walls in the same proportion, viz. 1:1:1:3.

thesis was maximal. During this process the rate of accumulation of glutamic acid varied inversely with the nucleic acid content. Penicillin, in common with another bactericidal antibiotic, bacitracin, had no effect upon the accumulation of free or combined glutamate in suspensions of resting bacteria but, when added to a growing culture, prevented the uptake of both. The work of Caldwell and Hinshelwood[33] had shown that nucleic acid guided the order of amino acids in protein synthesis in growing bacteria, while protein in turn guided the order of nucleotide synthesis. Hotchkiss had reported[34] that penicillin disorganised protein synthesis and led to an extracellular accumulation of peptides from the amino acids, though Gale's work showed that this would occur anyway if a complete mixture of amino acids was present. The role of penicillin was clearly dependent upon the amino acid composition of the medium. Also, Mitchell and Moyle[35], confirming the rise in intracellular nucleotides under the influence of penicillin, noted that

References p. 95/97

the expected rise in nucleic acid content of the cells during logarithmic growth was also prevented. If the primary biochemical disorder was an undue rise in nucleotides when cells were trying to grow in the presence of penicillin, there were also secondary disorders in the shape of defective synthesis of protein and nucleic acid related perhaps to another primary disorder affecting amino acid transportation into the cell. This would seem very likely if the binding site is the protoplast membrane, which is actively involved in transport and enzymatic work leading to protein synthesis[36].

Biochemical effects at different concentrations

These metabolic interferences by penicillin occurred at low concentrations which permitted a preliminary period of growth. At high concentrations different effects were obtained, both morphologically (see p. 83) and biochemically: it had already been claimed[37,38] that the primary effect of penicillin was inhibition of nucleic acid metabolism which is, of course, true of any organism which fails to divide. Gale, however, considered that the changes produced by high concentrations might be relevant to the development of resistance. Very high concentrations (2000 units/ml) corrected the acceleration of protein synthesis normally produced by the addition of purines and pyrimidines to bacteria suspended in glucose–amino acid mixtures. This again pointed to the connection between protein and nucleic acid synthesis. If penicillin, by interfering with amino acid transportation and protein synthesis, thereby affected the formation of nucleic acid, it might cause an altered nucleic acid to appear; he claimed also that, under these conditions, an adaptive penicillinase continued to be formed after removal of the penicillin and suggested that the altered nucleic acid produced indirectly by the penicillin might, by this and other means, transform sensitive into resistant cells. Another effect, observed[39] at lower concentrations (3–10 units/ml), was that penicillin, by inhibiting the incorporation of specific amino acid residues into the cell, blocked the orderly interaction of protein and nucleic acid, thereby stopping the synthesis of specific proteins. The β-galactosidase of staphylococci was also inhibited together with the synthesis of ribonucleic acid (RNA), irrespectively of whether RNA, DNA, purines or pyrimidines were present; these effects occurred at concentrations (1 unit/ml) which had no effect upon the catalase activity of staphylococci.

Studies on subcellular fractions

Had the Park nucleotides been concerned with nucleic acid synthesis, all this would have pointed to an effect by penicillin primarily upon nucleic acid metabolism, but this was far from being the case. The earlier biochemical studies had been made upon intact cells but the technique developed by Dawson[40], in which bacteria were shaken with minute glass beads in a sonic oscillator, permitted the cell and its wall to be separated. The cell wall of a gram-negative bacillus contained 11–20% lipid and a complete range of amino acids, whereas that of a gram-positive coccus contained only 2–4% lipid and fewer amino acids, none of which were aromatic. Cummins and Harris[41] found that all gram-positive walls examined contained a substance, muramic acid, which was soon to provide the clue to the riddle. This odd amino sugar, first characterised appropriately enough by Strange and Dark[42], proved to be a key compound in the structure of the mucopeptide polymer of all cell walls, in the form of the N-acetyl derivative. It was assigned the full name 3-O-α-carboxyethylglucosamine and soon synthesised[43,44].

Further studies on the cell wall during this time showed that lysozyme attacked the chemical bonds in the mucopeptide of some organisms[45], thereby removing the wall to leave the protoplast intact within the cytoplasmic membrane[46] which was entirely different in structure[47]. During multiplication of cells, all growth of the wall occurred outside this membrane[48]. Chemically, the wall of gram-positive bacteria consisted of glucosamine and N-acetylmuramic acid in a ratio of 1:1 joined to a peptide chain of DL-alanine, D-glutamic acid and either lysine or diaminopimelic acid[41]; a ribitol phosphate polymer was also present, linked to alanine and glucosamine to form a complex named teichoic acid[49]. Quantitative analysis of the cell wall showed that the amino sugar, glutamic acid, lysine and alanine were present in the ratio of 1:1:1:3, which was the ratio in which these substances were present in the Park nucleotide[50]. There was therefore a close similarity between part of the normal cell wall and the nucleotides which accumulated in the early stages in staphylococci treated with threshold concentrations of penicillin. There was also close agreement in the proportions of D-alanine and D-glutamic acid. This pointed to a unique biochemical process, since the complex D-alanine and 3-O-α-carboxyethylglucosamine was not found elsewhere, and D-glutamic acid was known to be rare. Park and Strominger[50] found that uridine nucleotide accumulated in penicillin-treated lactobacilli and β-haemolytic streptococci as well as in *Staph. aureus*; they therefore deduced that the nucleotide was a biosynthetic precursor of the cell wall

References p. 95/97

and that its accumulation in penicillin-treated cells was due to interference with its polymerisation to mucopeptide, possibly associated with an inhibition of transglycosidation.

There may also be interference with the other complex, teichoic acid, of the cell-wall mucopeptide. The base here is cytidine in place of uridine and the complete ribitol phosphate polymer may account for about half the dry weight of wall substance in some gram-positive organisms[49]. When *Staph. aureus* is treated with penicillin, cytidine diphosphate ribitol accumulates within the cell[51] and might represent the same sort of precursor-accumulation (to teichoic acid) as Park nucleotide.

Binding of penicillin within the cell

This explains in biochemical terms what penicillin does but not how or, in ultramicroscopic terms, where. The "lesion" is clearly interference with synthesis of cell-wall mucopeptide. The site might be the penicillin-binding component (PBC) of Rowley and Cooper[24]. This component is an ultra-microscopic lipid liberated by mechanical rupture of staphylococci; the disintegrated particles bind 7–12 times more penicillin than the intact cell[52]. PBC is lost when the particles, or the intact cells, are treated with a lipid-soluble substance such as phenol but not with anionic or cationic detergents[53] even when the latter cause cytolysis. The number of molecules of penicillin bound by PBC is quite small—of the order of 300 per intact cell—and most of the binding occurs very quickly before any biochemical changes can be detected[54]. Yet this minute degree of binding causes extensive metabolic consequences, leading to death of the bacterial cell. In contrast, penicillin is virtually non-toxic to non-bacterial cells, and lacks surface activity. The "lesion" must therefore occur at a strategic site which Cooper [55] suggested might be the osmotic barrier of the cell. From other studies, it is known that this is located in a lipid substance, close to the surface of the cell[56,57]. PBC has these properties and affects, as has been seen, cell-wall activities primarily: the particulate fraction contains phospholipid (10%), other lipids (10%) and a protein–glycerophosphate complex similar to that in the cell walls of gram-positive cocci[58]. Cooper found that penicillin was still bound by organisms trained to resistance, but Eagle[59] claimed that naturally-occurring resistant strains bound less penicillin, while other workers[60,61] have shown that the rate of uptake of penicillin by relatively resistant organisms such as *Bacillus cereus* and *Str. faecalis* is slower at any given concentration than the uptake by a sensitive *Staph. aureus*. Even so, most bacterial cells bind penicillin to some extent, and it is admitted[55] that the degree and rate of binding vary considerably under different experimental conditions *in vitro*.

Formation of spheroblasts and protoplasts

Most workers who have studied the mode of action of an antibacterial drug naturally select sensitive bacteria as test organisms and there is a tendency throughout this subject for general conclusions to be drawn from particular instances; anyone working at a bench in a clinical laboratory knows that the variations in sensitivity to antibiotics within a given species are sometimes as great as those between species. Such considerations must be applied critically to any deductions made about mode of action. There are few bacterial species which are not affected to some extent by penicillin, so studies on mode of action must be extended beyond the conventional list of sensitive species. Superficially, gram-negative bacilli appear to be resistant, but more critical studies, detailed earlier, show that penicillin causes striking changes in morphology and growth. *E. coli* is one such: at high concentrations, bacteriostasis and some lysis are produced by penicillin[19,62]. Lederberg[63] found that the addition of Mg ions and 10% sucrose permitted growth of this organism in the presence of penicillin but the cells were large, spherical and osmotically-sensitive due to the absence of a wall; these protoplasts reverted to normal when removed from penicillin which did not, however, have this effect on resting cells. The conclusion was that penicillin affected new cell-wall formation and not the existing cell wall[64]. Penicillin induces protoplast formation in *Proteus* as well as *E. coli*[65] and the resulting pattern of growth—as was noted by Fleming[66]—was very abnormal indeed. There is therefore a similarity of response between resistant gram-negative bacilli and sensitive gram-positive cocci in that abnormal swelling and then lysis, due to imperfect synthesis of the cell wall, can be produced by penicillin during growth. If the medium is rendered hypertonic by the addition of sucrose, the cell body withstands rupture, in staphylococci as in coliforms. The effect on the cell wall is therefore followed, as soon as the cell grows, by a secondary effect on the cytoplasmic lipid membrane which is a site of binding and which also controls osmosis and transport. This secondary effect would explain several of the other biochemical changes noted in penicillin-treated cells: the assimilation of amino acids; inhibition of β-galactosidase, a membrane enzyme[67]; and later effects on synthesis of protein and nucleic acid. If the membrane is preserved and the protoplast left intact in hypertonic sucrose, some of these effects are prevented; or, in the case of spheroblasts of resistant gram-negative bacilli, some degree of growth and metabolism continues with the formation of grotesque involutionary forms. The difference in susceptibility of gram-negative and gram-positive organisms to lysis, in hypotonic media, may be due to the rapidity with which the exposed cell body of the former loses small molecules[58] as well as to the lesser dependence, in the wall itself, upon nucleotide precursors for polymerisation into mucopeptide. Such a possibility is borne out by electron microscopy of penicillin-treated cells[68] by Canadian workers who conclude that "swelling, filamentous forms, large body formation, penicillin-insensitivity, L-forms of certain bacteria and lysis as morphological expressions of the effects of penicillin can be explained as interference with cell-wall synthesis and the consequent inability of the cell wall to act as an "osmotic corset" in a hypotonic environment." These studies, which were performed with methacrylate sections exposed to lanthanum nitrate to intensify the shadow of the cell wall, showed that the loss of density was most striking in the septum and that, if lysis was prevented by 0.3 M sucrose, the spheroblasts retained a cell wall but formed no septa. Penicillin-resistant staphylococci showed either no morphological change, or temporary damage to the septum when treated with penicillin. Recent studies have also shown that L-forms of staphylococci are highly resistant to penicillin G and methicillin in concentrations of 1000 μg/ml or more irrespectively of whether the parent cells are naturally sensitive or resistant[69]. It is also known that, in general, the parent cells of staphylococci are more sensitive to the bactericidal antibiotics penicillin, bacitracin and vancomycin[70], presumably because the cell wall is amenable to their interfering action, whereas protoplasts are more sensitive to the bacteriostatic antibiotics (tetracyclines, chloramphenicol and erythromycin) which appear to act variously on processes more likely to be located within the cell body[71].

Further studies on the chemistry of the cell wall

The N-acetyl derivative of muramic acid is now known to be present in the mucopeptide polymer of all bacterial cell walls and this probably explains the fact that penicillin always has some effect upon bacteria. In gram-positive cells, it is the key substance, though recent studies by Baddiley[49] and his associates attract increasing attention to the rival polymer teichoic acid which may be more important in some species than in others. Muramic acid was characterised and synthesised by Strange, Kent and others[42–44]. Stro-minger[72] approached the route of bacterial biosynthesis by incubating extracts of staphylococci and coliforms with labelled C-3 compounds in the presence of uridine diphosphate-N-acetylglucosamine. Of the compounds tested, only phosphoenolpyruvate would condense with the glycosamine nucleotide to give a C-3-substituted compound, thus:

$$\text{Phosphoenolpyruvate} + \text{ADP} \rightleftharpoons \text{pyruvate} + \text{ATP}$$

so that this substance is the likely precursor of the side-chain. This appears to be a self-sufficient system. Other workers[73–75] were finding that staphylococci could synthesise mucopeptide containing all the muramic acid available without synthesising protein. Some years before, Gale and Folkes[76] had noted that [^{14}C]aspartic acid labelled staphylococci during growth. Aspartic acid was not detectable in the cell wall[75], so it seemed that the labelling must be due to the incorporation of ^{14}C into the side-chain. This is supported by the more recent observation[77] that DL-alanine, pyruvate, lactate and aspartate all label the side-chain in preference to the pyranose ring of muramic acid. It is reported also that glucose is a precursor of all the carbon atoms in muramic acid under conditons favouring the synthesis of cell wall but not of protein[77]. Gram-negative bacilli contain very little mucopeptide in their cell walls[78] and it is now obvious that this in itself goes a long way toward explaining the lesser sensitivity of these organisms to penicillin though not to certain other antibiotics or to α- and p-aminopenicillanic acids (p. 101). Other mechanisms must therefore be involved and it may be that enzymes in the cytoplasmic membrane[79] concerned with protein synthesis in the cell wall (ref. 36, 80) are also affected, together with amino acid transportation across the cell wall, as outlined above. In this connection, Park[81] has confirmed the earlier observation by Gale that bactericidal antibiotics can inhibit the incorporation of amino acids into mucopeptide. The extent to which this relates to the specific binding of penicillin by the lipid or lipoprotein membrane[55] is uncertain. It seems likely that more than one enzyme system involved in wall synthesis may be disturbed, just as more than one type of precursor accumulates, even in sensitive gram-positive cocci[82]. Attention has also been drawn to the structural similarity between N-acetylmuramic acid and benzylpenicillin in respect of the steric location of their hydrogen-bonding groups[83] which might mean that penicillin is a competitive inhibitor to the incorporation of muramic acid in the mucopeptide.

References p. 95/97

MODE OF ACTION OF THE NEWER PENICILLINS

The foregoing account relates almost entirely to penicillin G. Very little attempt has been made to repeat in detail these elaborate biochemical and morphological studies upon organisms treated with the new derivatives of 6-APA though the need to do so, for fundamental as well as practical reasons, is imperative.

One reason for this is that, superficially, the pattern of activity shown by some of the new derivatives is very similar to that of penicillin G. Thus methicillin and the isoxazole penicillins, along with others possessing hindered side-chains, appear to act similarly upon staphylococci, causing lysis of rapidly-dividing cells at optimal concentrations. The activity of these derivatives against resistant staphylococci would seem to be explained by teric hindrance to the attachment of the enzyme. Yet this cannot be the full explanation. Many strains of *Staph. aureus* highly resistant to all forms of penicillin have now been described[84-88]; none of these strains has been shown convincingly to owe its resistance to inactivation of the newer derivatives, even though they are all strong penicillinase-formers. There is evidence[84-86], in some strains at least, that the resistant cells may constitute a different population which grows slowly and abnormally in the presence of methicillin; but there is also evidence that the resistance of staphylococci, whether natural or acquired, toward these new derivatives is qualitatively different from that exhibited toward penicillin G[85-87] even though it endows the organism with comparable resistance to all forms of penicillin.

Despite the similarity in general pattern, methicillin and the isoxazoles show a divergence from penicillin G in being much less active against streptococci and pneumococci and in being slower, though not necessarily less complete, in their lytic effect even upon staphylococci. If penicillin G acts upon all gram-positive cocci in the same way, by interference with cell-wall synthesis, then the newer derivatives do not; but, on staphylococci at least, their mode of action is said to be similar[89].

Even less is known about the mode of action of other derivatives which alter the antibacterial spectrum of penicillin in either direction. It must be accepted for the moment that there is a common mode of action, for resistance to one penicillin, whether natural or acquired, always seems to connote resistance either to the molecular analogues of that penicillin or even to the entire series of 6-APA derivatives. Apart from staphylococci, the inactivating enzymes amidase and β-lactamase also influence the sensitivity of coliforms (Chapter 13). Lastly, though perhaps first in importance, there are the structural differences in the penicillin molecules themselves, wherein a minor change can cause a major difference in intrinsic antibacterial properties. A study of the mode of action would be incomplete without detailed attention to structure–activity relationship, which will be considered in the next chapter.

REFERENCES

1 GARDNER, A. D., *Nature*, *146* (1940) 837.
2 HOBBY, G. L., MEYER, K. AND CHAFFEE, E., *Proc. Soc. exp. Biol. (N.Y.)*, *50* (1942) 281.
3 LEE, S. W., FOLEY, E. J. AND EPSTEIN, J. A., *J. Bact., 48* (1944) 393.
4 ABRAHAM, E. P., CHAIN, E., FLETCHER, C. M., FLOREY, H. W., GARDNER, A. D., HEATLEY, N. G. AND JENNINGS, M. A., *Lancet, ii* (1941) 177.
5 HOBBY, G. L., MEYER, K. AND CHAFFEE, E., *Proc. Soc. exp. Biol. (N.Y.)*, *50* (1942) 277.
6 RAMMELKAMP, C. A. AND KEEFER, C. S., *J. clin. Invest., 22* (1943) 649.
7 RAUG, L. A. AND KIRBY, W. M. M., *J. Immunol., 48* (1944) 335.
8 BIGGER, J. W., *Lancet, ii* (1944) 497.
9 GARROD, L. P., *Brit. med. J., I* (1945) 107.
10 KNOX, R., *Lancet, i* (1945) 559.
11 CHAIN, E. AND DUTHIE, E. S., *Lancet, i* (1945) 652.
12 TODD, E. W., *Lancet, i* (1945) 74.
13 STEWART, G. T., *Lancet, ii* (1945) 705.
14 THOMAS, A. R. AND LEVINE, M., *J. Bact., 49* (1945) 623.
15 DUGUID, J. P., *Edinb. med. J., 53* (1946) 401.
16 ERIKSEN, K. R., *Acta path. scand., 23* (1946) 3 (Sep.).
17 ØRSKOV, J., *J. Bact., 7* (1922) 537.
18 ERIKSEN, K. R., (1947) *Proceedings 4th international Congress Microbiol, Rosenkilde and Bagger, Copenhagen (1949)* p. 100.
19 STEWART, G. T., *J. Hyg. (Camb), 45* (1947) 282.
20 GALE, E. T. AND TAYLOR, E. S., *J. gen. Microbiol., 1* (1947) 314.
21 PARK, J. T. AND JOHNSON, M. J., *J. biol. Chem., 179* (1949) 585.
22 PARK, J. T., *Fed. Proc., 9* (1950) 213.
23 MAAS, E. A. AND JOHNSON, M. J., *J. Bact., 57* (1949) 415; *58* (1949) 361.
24 ROWLEY, D., COOPER, P. D., ROBERTS, P. W. AND LESTER SMITH, E., *Biochem. J., 46* (1950) 157.
25 GALE, E. F. AND RODWELL, A. W., *J. gen. Microbiol., 3* (1949) 127.
26 HOTCHKISS, R. D., *Advanc. Enzymol., 4* (1944) 153.
27 MCWUILLEN, K., *Symp. Soc. gen. Microbiol., 6* (1956) 127.
28 PARK, J. T., *J. biol. Chem., 194* (1952) 877.
29 PARK, J. T., *J. biol. Chem., 194* (1952) 885.
30 PARK, J. T., *J. biol. Chem., 194* (1952) 897.
31 GALE, E. F., *Biochem. J., 48* (1951) 290.
32 GALE, E. F. AND FOLKES, JOAN P., *Biochem. J., 53* (1953) 483.
33 CALDWELL, P. C. AND HINSHELWOOD, C., *J. chem. Soc., 3151* (1950) 3156.
34 HOTCHKISS, R. D., *J. exp. Med., 91* (1950) 351.
35 MITCHELL, P. D. AND MOYLE, J., *J. gen. Microbiol., 5* (1951) 421.
36 BUTLER, J. A. V., CRATHORN, A. R. AND HUNTER, G. D., *Biochem. J., 69* (1958) 544.
37 KRAMPITZ, L. O. AND WERKMAN, C. H., *Arch. Biochem., 12* (1947) 57.
38 GROS, F. AND MACHEBŒUF, M., *Ann. Inst. Pasteur, 74* (1948) 308.

39 GALE, E. F., *Nature, 173* (1954) 1223.
40 DAWSON, J. M., *Symp. Soc. gen. Microbiol, 1* (1949) 119.
41 CUMMINS, C. S. AND HARRIS, H., *J. gen. Microbiol., 14* (1956) 583.
42 STRANGE, R. E. AND DARK, F. A., *Nature, 177* (1956) 186.
43 STRANGE, R. E. AND KENT, L. H., *Biochem. J., 71* (1959) 733.
44 ZILLIKEN, F., *Fed. Proc., 18* (1959) 966.
45 WEIBULL, C., *J. Bact., 66* (1952) 688.
46 WEIBULL, C., *Exp. Cell Res., 10* (1956) 214.
47 ROBINOW, C. F. AND MURRAY, R. G. E., *Exp. Cell Res.*, (1953) 390.
48 DAWSON, J. M. AND STERN, H., *Biochim. biophys. Acta (Amst.), 13* (1954) 31.
49 ARMSTRONG, J. J., BADDILEY, J., BUCHANAN, J. C., CARSS, B. AND GREENBERG, G. R., *J. chem. Soc.*, (1958) 4344.
50 PARK, J. T. AND STROMINGER, J. C., *Science, 125* (1957) 99.
51 BUCHANAN, J. G., GREENBERG, G. R., CARSS, B., ARMSTRONG, J. J. AND BADDILEY, J., (1958) *Internat. Congress of Biochemistry, Vienna 1–6 Sept.*, 1958, p. 7.
52 COOPER, P. D., *J. gen. Microbiol., 10* (1954) 236.
53 COOPER, P. D., *Biochim. biophys. Acta (Amst.), 13* (1954) 433.
54 COOPER, P. D., *J. gen. Microbiol., 13* (1954) 22.
55 COOPER, P. D., *Bact. Rev., 20* (1956) 28.
56 WORK, T. S. AND WORK, E., *Basis of Chemotherapy*, Oliver and Boyd, Edinburgh and London, 1948, p. 234.
57 MITCHELL, P., *Symp. Soc. gen. Microbiol., 1* (1949) 55.
58 MITCHELL, P. AND MOYLE, J., *J. gen. Microbiol., 10* (1954) 533.
59 EAGLE, H., *J. exp. Med., 99* (1954) 207.
60 REYNOLDS, BETTY AND ROWLEY, D., *Brit. J. exp. Path., 34* (1953) 651.
61 POLLOCK, M. R., *Brit. J. exp. Path., 34* (1953) 251.
62 LEDERBERG, J., *J. Bact., 73* (1957) 144.
63 LEDERBERG, J., *Proc. Nat. Acad. Sci. (Wash.), 42* (1956) 574.
64 HAHN, F. E. AND CIAK, J., *Science, 125* (1957) 119.
65 PEASE, P., *J. gen. Microbiol., 17* (1957) 64.
66 FLEMING, A., VOUREKA, A., KRAMER, I. R. H. AND HUGHES, W. H., *J. gen. Microbiol., 4* (1950) 257.
67 CREASER, E. R., *J. gen. Microbiol., 12* (1955) 288.
68 MURRAY, R. G. E., FRANCOMBE, W. H. AND MAYALL, B. H., *Canad. J. Microbiol., 5* (1959) 641.
69 KAGAN, B. M., MARTIN, E. R. AND STEWART, G. T., *Nature, 203* (1964) 1031.
70 KAGAN, B. M., MOLANDER, C. W., HEIMLICH, H. J., ZOLLA, SUSAN AND LIEPNIEKS, SILVYA, *Abstract of 3rd Interscience Conference on Antimicrobial Agents and Chemotherapy, Washington, Oct. 28–30*, 1963, p. 63.
71 GALE, E. F., *Brit. med. Bull., 16* (1960) 11.
72 STROMINGER, J. C., *Biochim. biophys. Acta, 30* (1958) 645.
73 MANDELSTAM, J. AND ROGERS, H. J., *Nature, 181* (1958) 956.
74 HANCOCK, R. AND PARK, J. T., *Nature, 181* (1958) 1050.
75 MANDELSTAM, J. AND ROGERS, H. J., *Biochem. J., 72* (1959) 654.
76 GALE, E. F. AND FOLKES, JOAN P., *Biochem. J., 55* (1953) 721.
77 RICHMOND, M. H. AND PERKINS, H. R., *Biochem. J., 85* (1962) 580.
78 MANDELSTAM, J., *Nature, 189* (1961) 855.
79 MITCHELL, P. D. AND MOYLE, J., *Biochem. J., 64* (1956) 19.
80 CRATHORN, A. R. AND HUNTER, G. D., *Biochem. J., 69* (1958) 47.
81 PARK, J. T., *Biochem. J., 71* (1958) 2.
82 SAUKONNEN, J. J., *Nature, 192* (1961) 816.
83 COLLINS, J. F. AND RICHMOND, M. H., *Nature, 195* (1962) 142.

[84] JEVONS, M. PATRICIA, *Brit. med. J.*, *I* (1961) 124 (corresp.).
[85] STEWART, J. T., *Brit. med. J.*, *I* (1961) 863.
[86] BARBER, MARY AND WATERWORTH, PAMELA M., *Brit. med. J.*, *I* (1962) 1159.
[87] STEWART, G. T. AND HOLT, R. J., *Brit. med. J.*, *I* (1963) 308.
[88] ERIKSEN, K. R., AND ERICHSEN, I., *Brit. med. J.*, *I* (1963) 746.
[89] ROGERS, H. AND JELIASEWICZ, J., *Biochem. J.*, *81* (1961) 576.

Chapter 10

THE MODE OF ACTION OF PENICILLINS. II

STRUCTURE–ACTIVITY RELATIONSHIPS

The intention here is to consider changes in intrinsic antibacterial activity wrought by accidental or deliberate modification of the penicillin molecule; purely pharmacological changes which may also be produced thereby are ignored in this chapter.

EARLY STUDIES

Elucidation of the structure of the natural penicillins was no easy matter, even when purified extracts had been obtained. Purified material, in short supply until 1944, was unstable and urgently required for clinical purposes, so that elaborate chemical studies were extremely difficult. The presence of sulphur in the molecule was not known until July 1943 (refs. 1 and 2); by the end of 1943, penicilloic acid was identified as an inert product of degradation and it was clear that biological activity resided in an unknown closed-ring anhydride of penicilloic acid. It was considered then by all the Anglo-American authorities that the ring must be of thiazolidine–oxazolone structure which the organic chemists should have been able to synthesise in a month or two; the true lactam–thiazolidine structure eluded identification until 1945 (ref. 3). By this time it was known that addition of phenyl-acetate as a precursor in the brew increased activity by favouring biosynthesis of benzylpenicillin, but that antibacterial activity could also be obtained with various other side-chains.

The natural penicillins thus identifiable varied considerably in intrinsic antibacterial activity, thus:

	Oxford units/mg
Penicillin F	1550
Penicillin G	1667
Penicillin K (*n*-heptyl-)	2300
Penicillin X (*p*-hydroxybenzyl-)	900

The higher activity of penicillin K was offset by excessive protein binding. The consistently high activity of penicillin G against pyogenic cocci made it the penicillin of choice, but the only available structural variant, the *p*-hydroxybenzylpenicillin X, had lower activity[4], though it was later found that azo derivatives of this were more active against *Staph. aureus*[5]. Most other derivatives prepared during these years were much less active than the natural penicillins, with the possible exception of the phenylmercaptyl, which is reported to be more active against streptococci[6].

The next indication of an important structural modification came from cephalosporin N (Penicillin N, synnematin B). This substance has an α-aminoadipyl side-chain, and is now known to be D-4-amino-4-carboxybutyl penicillin. The Oxford workers[7] found that the presence of the α-amino instead of the benzyl side-chain was associated with a hundredfold loss in activity against *Staph. aureus* but with higher activity against coliform bacilli. Acylation of the free amino group restored some of the activity against gram-positive organisms[8]. A few years later, Canadian workers[9] observed the same trend when they made *p*-aminobenzyl penicillin, which displayed considerable heightening of activity against coliform and other gram-negative bacilli; *N*-acylation again diverted the antibacterial spectrum toward the gram-positive pattern though, with the *p*-aminobenzyl derivative, the original loss of such activity was much less than with the α-aminoadipyl structure. These biochemical routes toward altered activity were selected by Chain and the Beecham workers[10] for their early experiments and, had it not been for the isolation of 6-APA, might have become the principal means of modifying the penicillin molecule.

None of the molecular modifications described above produced a penicillin of therapeutic utility, though it is possible that a well-designed clinical trial might have disclosed advantages in penicillin N (cephalosporin N) or *p*-aminobenzyl penicillin in virtue of their activity against gram-negative bacilli. The only modification which led to a therapeutic penicillin was the introduction of a polar group in the side-chain, to give phenoxymethyl penicillin (penicillin V). This compound attained importance solely by reason of its acid-stability, for the spectrum was slightly narrower than that of penicillin G and the intrinsic activity lower.

6-AMINOPENICILLANIC ACID

The isolation of this substance[11] which is the molecular nucleus of all natural and semi-synthetic penicillins has made possible any number of systematic modifications of the side-chain. At present, and as far as is known, improvement in antibacterial activity can only occur by acylation in the 6-position, thus:

$$R—CO—HN—\underset{6}{CH}———\overset{S}{\underset{5}{CH}}\;\;\overset{}{\underset{2}{C}}—(CH_3)_2$$

The side-chains must be linked to the fused β-lactam–thiazolidine ring structure of 6-APA by a peptide linkage. The introduction of various side-chains R (Table VIII) has already yielded several penicillins of different therapeutic properties and many more with new biological properties, also of considerable theoretical interest. Since the penicillin molecule can be regarded as a fusion of two amino acids, L-cysteine and L-valine (Fig. 2), it follows that all derivatives prepared by substitution in the 6-position are acyl dipeptides. In mode of action, particularly in so far as they cause lysis by inhibition of cell-wall synthesis as described in the preceding chapter, the penicillins share

TABLE VIII

FACTORIAL INCREASE IN ACTIVITY OF 6-AMINOPENICILLANIC ACID PRODUCED BY THE PRESEN
OF IMPORTANT SIDE-CHAINS

Side chain (R)	Name of derivative	Increase in activity against					
		Staph. aureus		Str. pyogenes	Esch. coli	S. typhi	Klebsie
		Oxford	P'ase				
CH—CO—	Benzyl (G)	2500	Decrease	10000	None	20	None
CH₃O / —CO— / CH₃O	Methicillin	25	100	100	Decrease	Decrease	Decreas
—CH—CH—CO (N, C, O)	Oxacillin	500	2500	1000	Decrease	Decrease	Decreas
CH—CO— / NH₂	Ampicillin	1000	Decrease	5000	10	50	2
NH₂ / COOH —CH—CH—CO—	Penicillin (Cephalosporin) N	None	Decrease	50	5	10	None

features with other peptide or polypeptide antibiotics, such as bacitracin and polymyxin, which are structurally very different.

Antibacterial properties of 6-APA

6-APA inhibits pyogenic gram-positive bacteria thus:

Organism	MIC (µg/ml)
Staph. aureus	60–70
Staph. aureus (penicillinase)	> 200
Streptococci group A	50–100
Streptococci group D	> 200
Corynebacterium spp.	1–5
Sarcina lutea	30–50

It is therefore about 2000–10,000 times less active than benzyl penicillin against representative gram-positive organisms with the exception of *Corynebacterium*[12]. It is, however, not devoid of activity against gram-negative bacilli, thus:

	MIC (µg/ml)
Esch. coli	50–100
Aerobacter aerogenes	100–500
Proteus spp.	50–250
Salmonella spp.	50
Shigella spp.	50

These figures indicate that it possesses the same (low) order of activity as penicillin G against certain coliforms, though it has only about a tenth to a twentieth of the activity against some species of *Proteus* and against *Salmonella*. As with cephalosporin N and *p*-aminobenzyl penicillin, the possession of a free amino group confers activity, to some extent preferentially, against gram-negative bacilli and *N*-acylation restores the gram-positive spectrum. This is the general trend with penicillins, though there are exceptions which may be important: *p*-aminobenzyl penicillin is by no means inactive *per se* against gram-positive organisms, while 6-APA is more active than penicillin G against *chromobacterium*[12]. For practical purposes, however, the intrinsic antibacterial activity of 6-APA is very low indeed; useful activity is obtained only by acylation[13], the degree and width of activity being determined by the nature of the side-chain. In all known modifications, the 6-APA ring-structure must remain intact, since breakage at any point leads to complete loss of antibacterial activity, irrespectively of the side-chain. The action of 6-APA is bactericidal at the minimum inhibitory concentration or slightly above: it produces the same morphological changes as penicillin G on partially sensitive gram-negative bacilli and may be presumed therefore also to inhibit cell-wall synthesis[12].

It must be remembered that, even in the crystalline state, 6-APA may contain other substances of a penicillin-like nature. Batchelor, Rolinson and their colleagues[14] noted the presence of two additional substances with weak antibacterial activity but not identifiable chromatographically as known penicillins. Factor 1 was present in all preparations of 6-APA, whether obtained by fermentation with *Penicillium chrysogenum*, or by enzymatic hydrolysis of penicillins G or V. This factor showed greater activity against gram-positive organisms than 6-APA but less activity against gram-negative bacilli; if present in concentrations of about 2% in the 6-APA, it could conceivably account for all the gram-positive activity of the compound. Factor 2 was present in greater quantity but had lower antibacterial activity. A third factor was also detected, with high activity against gram-positive organisms, but could not be separated from factors 1 and 2. All the factors were dialysable which differentiated them from the complex poly-6-APA described by Grant *et al.*[15]. At the time of writing there is no further information on the nature of these factors.

Systematic modification of 6-APA

α-phenoxyalkyl derivatives

The first compounds to be prepared and studied in detail were the alkyl derivatives of phenoxymethyl penicillin substituted in the α-position[16]. This was an obvious lead to follow, since α-substitution was known to bring acid stability. It was also found that, as the side-chain became larger, the activity against penicillin-sensitive *Staph. aureus* decreased, though some derivatives showed a relative increase of activity against penicillinase-forming staphylococci due to greater stability toward the inactivating enzyme. This was maximal with α-phenoxyisobutyl penicillin. It is now known that increasing chain-length is accompanied by a fall in activity not only against staphylococci but against all other penicillin-sensitive organisms, and also by a narrowing in spectrum. Protein binding also increases.

These derivatives have the following general structure in the side-chain:

$$R - \langle\bigcirc\rangle - O-CH-CO-NH$$
$$\underset{CH_3(CH_2)_n}{|}$$

All compounds of this series have an asymmetric carbon atom and have been examined usually as diastereoisomeric mixtures though with some derivatives one isomer may be more active than the other. This line of investigation led to the introduction of phenethicillin and propicillin as therapeutic substances (Chapter 4) with marginal pharmacological advantages. The other phenoxyalkyl derivatives are of theoretical interest only at present, though the differences in activity between these closely related compounds and their isomers merit close study. Against large inocula of penicillinase-forming staphylococci, the isobutyl derivative is about ten times as active as the butyl, whereas the isopropyl is only slightly more active than the propyl derivative[16]. The most important substitution in the α-position from the practical viewpoint is with a free amino group, giving ampicillin (pp. 46, 100).

Substitution in the phenyl group

The α-phenoxyalkyl modifications described above affected the intermediate part of the side-chain and its length. There are greater opportunities for substitution in the terminal benzene ring, or in total replacement of the phenylacetyl side-chain, Doyle, Nayler and their colleagues have achieved this by treating 6-APA with acylating agents[17], usually acid chlorides, thus:

$$N-CH-\underset{|}{CH}\overset{S}{\diagdown}C-(CH_3)_2 \quad + \; R-CO-Cl \rightarrow \quad R-CONH-CH-\underset{|}{CH}\overset{S}{\diagdown}C-(CH_3)_2 \; +HCl$$
$$\underset{O}{\diagup}C-N-CH-COOH \qquad\qquad\qquad \underset{O}{\diagup}C-N-CH-COOH$$

They found that trisubstituted methyl penicillins were more stable toward penicillinase, especially when all three substituents were "fairly bulky", and suggested that steric hindrance around the side-chain amide linkage prevented attachment to the active sites of the enzyme. Thus triphenylmethyl penicillin (R = Ph$_3$C), an analogue of penicillin G, was stable, whereas the diphenylmethyl analogue (R = Ph$_2$CH) was inactivated by staphylococcal penicillinase. This trend led Doyle and Nayler[18] to try side-chains prepared from sterically-hindered carboxylic acids. It was found that steric hindrance operated around the side-chain amide linkage with 2,6-disubstituted phenyl-penicillins; phenylpenicillin itself was unstable to penicillinase and weak in antibacterial potency. Various 2,6-dialkoxyphenylpenicillins were however relatively resistant to the enzyme. The outstanding example was 2,6-dimethoxyphenylpenicillin (methicillin) $[R = Ph(CH_3O)_2]$. The 2,4-dimethoxyphenylpenicillin was inactivated by penicillinase, confirming the likelihood that resistance to the enzyme was steric in origin around the amide linkage. Further increase in molecular weight of these 2,6-dialkoxybenzoyl derivatives led to a sharp lessening in antibacterial activity. This was found also by Gourevitch et al.[19] who noted a relationship between increasing molecular weight and serum binding. N-substituted phthalamic acids are also moderately active and stable to penicillinase[20].

Analogues of methicillin were prepared by incorporating side-chains consisting of sterically-hindered alkoxynaphthoic and quinolinecarboxylic acids[21], giving various naphthyl and quinolyl derivatives which were relatively stable to penicillinase. One such derivative, 6-(2-ethoxynaphthamido)-penicillanic acid (nafcillin) has now been produced by Wyeth[22] as a therapeutic substance with a spectrum of activity very similar to the isoxazole penicillins but with poor oral absorption[23] and probably a lower order of therapeutic activity (p. 42).

A series of quinoline and quinoxaline derivatives has also been studied[24], some of which are also active against staphylococci and resistant to penicillinase. One compound, 3-carboxy-2-quinoxalinyl penicillin (quinacillin) is selectively active against staphylococci and highly resistant to penicillinase. Quinolines and quinoxalines possess antibacterial activity per se; it is known that some halogenated oxy- and hydroxyquinolines[25] and certain quinoxaline-N-dioxides are relatively active against some gram-negative bacilli. Curiously enough, the presence of this type of side-chain in penicillin does not seem to broaden activity to any appreciable extent; indeed, quinacillin has a very narrow spectrum (p. 43). The effect of further substitution in this side-chain, especially halogenation, might merit attention.

The activity and steric hindrance of methicillin depend upon the presence of two methoxy groups on the benzene ring. No advantages appeared to be conferred by substitution with electron-attracting groups elsewhere in the ring[26]. Increasing strength of the side-chain acids led to greater acid stability but usually to lower antibacterial activity. This applies to derivatives with two, one or no methoxy groups, and also to halogenated derivatives. The most successful modification of the side-chain in this direction is represented by the various isoxazoles (p. 38) which are stable to acid and staphylococcal penicillinase, and show higher intrinsic activity than methicillin against other pyogenic cocci besides staphylococci[27]. There is reason to believe also that halogenation increases the activity of these derivatives, as in cloxacillin and its analogues[28]. In pursuit of this effect, a number of other side-chains have also been tested, including halo-alkyl[29], and the products of reaction with cyanates and cyclic anhydrides[30]. 2-biphenylyl penicillin showed promise[31] but is now known to produce lower blood levels and to be less active than the isoxazoles.

Substitution in and around the phenyl side-chain of 6-APA is therefore of paramount importance in limiting hydrolysis by β-lactamase. Recent studies (Chapter 16) indicate that the side-chains of derivatives of 7-amino ce-phalosporanic acid (7-ACA) likewise affect the susceptibility of this form of lactam ring structure to hydrolysis, but also reveal, more clearly with 7-ACA than with 6-APA, that there are further important differences according to the source of the enzyme. The presence of a phenyl configuration in the N-acyl derivatives of both compounds greatly increases affinity for β-lact-amase from staphylococci though hydrolysis is, of course, limited if the side-chain is hindered. A charged α-amino-adipyl side-chain lessens susceptibility of 6-APA and 7-ACA to β-lactamase from *B. cereus* as well as from staphy-lococci; irrespectively of the side-chain configuration, the lactam-dihydro-thiazine ring of 7-ACA is intrinsically more stable to most forms of β-lact-amase, including those from coliforms, than the lactam-thiazolidine of 6-APA. This points to a route for synthesising β-lactam antibiotics with greater potency against penicillinase-forming gram-negative bacilli.

The derivatives of 6-APA at present available fall into three categories in terms of their susceptibility to β-lactamase. The susceptible derivatives (penicillin G, penicillin V, ampicillin, p-aminobenzyl penicillin) have high affinity with low Michaelis constant (K_m) and are rapidly hydrolysed at high substrate concentrations. These derivatives are more active than any others against non-penicillinase forming organisms. At the other extreme, the deriv-atives with hindered side-chains have a high K_m, with lesser affinity, and a much lower rate of hydrolysis. This group, therefore, inhibits resistant and sensitive staphylococci at about the same concentrations. The intermediate group includes the α-phenoxy-ethyl (phenethicillin) and higher derivatives with a high K_m and relatively high rate of hydrolysis. It is possible, there-fore, to classify penicillins, almost predictably, in terms of their high, intermediate or low susceptibility to β-lactamase. The relationship of this variable to three others is shown in Table X.

The immediate practical outcome of this knowledge is a series of penicillins stable to β-lactamase in varying degree. The gain may, in the long run, be more important if stability to other forms of β-lactamase can be combined with the wider activity which can now be glimpsed in some other derivatives of 6-APA and 7-ACA. Short of this, the advance in enzymology emanating from the wide range of β-lactam substrates now available is by no means negligible.

BROADENING OF ANTIBACTERIAL SPECTRUM

None of the numerous derivatives mentioned above has widened the activity of the penicillins. This has so far been achieved only by the introduction of free amino groups, in the following compounds:

R =

(1)   H$_2$N \>CH—CH$_2$CH$_2$CH$_2$CO—   D-4-amino-4-carboxy-*n*-butyl[32] (cephalo-
        HOOC   sporin N, synnematin B)

(2)   H$_2$N⟨ ⟩—CH$_2$CO—   *p*-aminobenzyl[9]

(3)   ⟨ ⟩—CH—CO—
              |
              NH$_2$ D(—) or L(+) α-aminobenzyl (ampicillin)

Of these three substances (1) is of natural origin, (2) and (3) are prepared biosynthetically. The antibacterial activity of (1) against gram-positive organisms is relatively low but it has more activity against *Salmonella* and other gram-negative bacilli. The side-chain is derived from the highly polar D-α-aminoadipic acid; the substance is optically active and more hydrophilic than most penicillins. Acylation of the free amino group endows the molecule with gram-positive activity[33].

Substances (2) (ref. 9) and (3) (refs. 33 and 34) retain activity slightly less than that of penicillin G against gram-positive bacteria and are more active against a fairly wide range of gram-negative bacilli, including all *Salmonellae*, many strains of *Proteus* and coliforms. With substitution at the α-carbon atom, ampicillin is acid stable. Both substances have an unusually high degree of activity against enterococci[35], including streptococci of group D, but both are susceptible to penicillinases from various sources. Substances (2) and (3) derive their wider activity entirely from the introduction of the reactive basic NH$_2$ group into the molecule of benzyl penicillin; this was a logical step in deliberate structural modification, since it was known that *N*-acylation of 4-aminobenzylpenicillin[9] as well as of cephalosporin N caused some reversion toward the gram-positive pattern of activity. Several other penicillins with amino-substituted side-chains have also been prepared[36] but there is no indication as yet that any of these are as active as ampicillin, which induces spheroblasts readily in *E. coli*[37] and appears to have a type of activity very similar to that of penicillin G.

FURTHER STERIC CONSIDERATIONS

The importance of steric hindrance to the attachment of the enzyme β-lactamase has already been discussed in detail. Similar hindrance may also limit the susceptibility of some penicillins to amidase, which has much less effect upon methicillin and the isoxazoles than upon penicillins G or V (p. 145). Steric factors affect also the action of several other penicillins on account of asymmetry of their molecules. Thus ampicillin shows higher activity, especially against gram-negative bacilli, in the D(−) than in the L(+) isomer[34]. The same applies to the D-isomer of α-hydroxybenzyl penicillin but not to phenethicillin, whose L-isomer is the more active.

These apparent anomalies are explained by the work of the Bristol group[38] who compared Fischer–Rosanoff projections if the side-chain precursors of various optically-active derivatives of 6-APA in relation to a fixed position of the asymmetric carbon atom. This showed similarity in the positions of the carboxyl, phenyl and remaining substituent of L-α-phenoxypropionic acid in relation to D-α-amino- and D-α-hydroxyphenylacetic acids. Molecular models revealed the same spatial relationship if the molecule was orientated in respect of the bulky (phenyl or phenoxy) group in the side-chain.

If the antibacterial activity of penicillin depends upon binding to a specific site within the organism, these and other steric factors must play a part in the process. Since it is clear that the degree and nature of activity of all penicillins are governed by the side-chain, it would appear that the similarity in structural relationship of the more active isomers of the compounds mentioned above provides an example of the kind of spatial configuration which is most amenable to binding. At the same time, it should be remembered that there are differences—as well as similarities—between the mode of action of penicillins upon gram-negative bacilli and gram-positive cocci, and that binding has been studied adequately only in the latter.

GRADING OF ACTIVITY

The highest intrinsic activity against the common pathogens is exhibited at the time of writing by three penicillins—penicillin G, ampicillin and cloxacillin (Table IX). In this respect, ampicillin is to a large extent complementary to penicillin G, for there are few organisms inhibited by one which are not to some extent affected also by the other. Cloxacillin enters the table only by reason of its high activity against penicillinase-forming staphylococci, though its effect upon some other pyogenic cocci is by no means negligible.

In terms of practical therapeutics, therefore, the structure-activity relationships described in this chapter yield a smaller dividend than might be expected. Penicillin G remains the penicillin with the highest degree of intrinsic activity against sensitive organisms. The addition of the free amino group in ampicillin heightens activity against certain gram-negative bacilli but in no way overcomes the susceptibility of the molecule to penicillinases. The hindered side-chain of cloxacillin interferes with the action of penicillinase from staphylococci and renders these organisms uniformly sensitive. The

TABLE IX

THERAPEUTIC PENICILLINS SHOWING MAXIMUM ACTIVITY
AGAINST REPRESENTATIVE BACTERIA

Organism	Maximal activity		Reservations
	Large inoculum	Small inoculum	
Staph. aureus	Penicillin G		
Staph. aureus (penicillinase)	Cloxacillin	Penicillin G	
Streptococcus group A	Penicillin G		
Streptococcus group D	Ampicillin		
Streptococcus other groups	Penicillin G or Ampicillin		Some are resistant to
Streptococcus viridans	Penicillin G or Ampicillin		Penicillin G
Streptococcus anaerobic	Penicillin G or Ampicillin		
Pneumococcus	Penicillin G		
Meningococcus	Penicillin G		
Gonococcus	Penicillin G		Occasionally resistant
C. diphtheriae	Penicillin G		
B. anthracis	Penicillin G		
Clostridia spp.	Penicillin G		
Haemophilus spp.	Ampicillin		cf. Phenylmercaptyl-
E. coli	Ampicillin		penicillin
K. aerogenes	Ampicillin		Many strains resistant
P. mirabilis	Ampicillin		Mainly resistant
P. vulgaris	Ampicillin		
Salmonella spp.	Ampicillin		
Actinomyces spp.	Penicillin G		

fact that substitution occurs at the α-carbon in both ampicillin and cloxacillin—in common with several other derivatives—makes these drugs acid stable and suitable for oral administration. Despite the immense effort now being made in the biosynthetic field, there is no evidence that any further radical changes in antibacterial properties of compounds modelled upon 6-APA have been effected, nor have the reasons for the resistance of *Mycobacteria, Ps. pyocyanea, Bacterium aerogenes* and many strains of coliforms and *Proteus* been uncovered.

STRUCTURE IN RELATION TO CHANGES IN BACTERIA

The morphological changes produced in bacteria by penicillin G have also been noted, less widely, with 6-APA and ampicillin acting upon gram-negative bacilli. Several of the newer derivatives however are entirely inert toward gram-negative bacilli; these derivatives include methicillin, the isoxazoles, the α-phenoxyalkyl penicillins and, in general terms, those which present steric hindrance to enzymatic hydrolysis. To explain this, Knox[39] has suggested that gram-negative bacilli have a receptor surface which is attacked only when closely in contact with one of the side-chains attached to the carbon next to the aromatic ring. This being the site where steric hindrance to enzyme-attachment operates most effectively, the very property which endows the molecule with activity against resistant staphylococci makes it ineffective against gram-negative bacilli. According to Knox, the site of gram-positive activity resides in the side-chain between the "gram-negative site" and the lactam ring, probably involving the carbonyl group. The activity of a hindered side-chain against gram-positive organisms is therefore preserved. This hypothesis offers an unusual diagrammatic sketch—or cartoon—of the mode of action of penicillins but, as Knox admits: "It must inevitably be inaccurate in part". It does not explain the high resistance of organisms which are morphologically altered by contact with penicillin, nor the relatively low intrinsic activity of some hindered penicillins, like quinacillin, against most gram-positive organisms; nor does it account for the high gram-negative activity possessed by cephalosporin N and *p*-aminobenzyl penicillin, with reactive groups far removed from the "gram-negative site". On the other hand, the hypothesis undoubtedly raises a logical query as to what is the molecular site of binding. This points to the need for further studies, on the lines laid by Rowley, Maas and Cooper, on the uptake of various labelled derivatives of 6-APA by sensitive and less sensitive organisms. In view of the profound effect of the side-chain upon activity, and the diversity of side-chains now available, it may be that totally different modes of action are operating. This has already been suggested[40] in the case of cephalosporin N which, with an amino acid side-chain, can form a zwitterion different in biological properties from the phenylacetic acid side-chains. The presence of additional amino-acids and of 6-APA itself is reported[41] to favour the lysis of *Esch. coli* by both isomers of ampicillin. It may be presumed—though it is by no means proved—that derivatives like ampicillin[37] which cause swelling, elongation and lysis, similar to that observed with penicillin G, act also by inhibiting mucopeptide synthesis in the cell wall; but, even if this is so, and even if inactivating enzymes are taken into account, the activity and lack of activity of the newer derivatives in certain directions still await explanation.

One major factor which limits the credibility of all existing hypotheses about mode of action is the variation in sensitivity within certain single species of bacteria. This applies especially to certain gram-negative bacilli, such as *E. coli* and *Proteus*, and to a lesser extent to gram-positive cocci which tend to show more uniform behaviour, with the exception of entero-cocci and *Str. viridans*. This variation, which has to be differentiated from that due to the inactivating enzymes amidase and β-lactamase formed by some gram-negative bacilli (Chapter 13), can be observed with seemingly identical organisms. For instance, some strains of *Esch. coli* are inhibited by penicillin G at 20 μg/ml, while others require 200 μg/ml. These differences have been studied in relation to enzyme production[42,43] but not to other biochemical factors such as accumulation of nucleotide precursors. Since the validity of the existing biochemical hypotheses depends largely upon the differences observed between a few strains of gram-positive cocci and even fewer strains of gram-negative bacilli, it is obviously important to see if like differences occur between non-penicillinase-forming resistant and less re-sistant gram-negative bacilli and enterococci. In this respect, some of the structure–activity relationships are consistent: all gram-negative bacilli and enterococci are resistant to derivatives with hindered side-chains, such as methicillin and the isoxazoles; as a class and with certain important excep-tions, these organisms tend to be such less resistant to the unhindered side-chains (Table X). There is therefore a negative correlation between insuscep-tibility to penicillinase and activity against gram-negative bacilli, but a posi-tive correlation between such activity and the presence of free amino groups in the side-chain. This applies also to the other peptide antibiotics poly-myxin and circulin which have 5–6 basic groups and attack gram-negative

TABLE X

SCHEMATIC PATTERN OF SENSITIVITY OF BACTERIA TO THE MAIN
THERAPEUTIC PENICILLINS

Side-chain of 6-APA	Intrinsic antibacterial effect on		Susceptibility to enzymes	
	Gram-negative bacilli	Gram-positive cocci*	Penamidase	β-lactamase
Dimethoxybenzyl Phenylisoxazolyl Phenoxyethyl Phenoxypropyl	Minimal	Intermediate	Minimal	Minimal
Phenoxymethyl Benzyl	Intermediate	Maximal	Maximal	maximal
α-aminobenzyl p-aminobenzyl	Maximal	maximal	Intermediate	Maximal

* Excluding β-lactamase-forming staphylococci.

bacilli, whereas those with fewer basic groups or none, such as tyrocidin and etamycin[44] attack only gram-positive organisms. The presence of a basic free amino group at various positions in the side-chain must therefore be a key factor in gram-negative activity; but it does not, like some other substituents, lead to a loss of gram-positive activity provided the side-chain is of benzyl structure.

REFERENCES

[1] ABRAHAM, E. P., CHAIN, E., BAKER, W. AND ROBINSON, R., Nature, 151 (1943) 107.
[2] ALICINO, J. F., Arch. Biochem., 27 (1950) 221.
[3] See The Chemistry of Penicillin, CLARKE, H. T., JOHNSON, J. R. AND ROBINSON, R. (Eds.), Princeton University Press, 1949.
[4] LIBBY, R. L. AND HOLMBERG, N. L., Science, 102 (1945) 303.
[5] FLOREY, H. W., et al. Antibiotics, Oxford University Press, 1949.
[6] McCARTHY, C. G., WALLMARK, G. AND FINLAND, M., Amer. J. med. Sci., 241 (1961) 143.
[7] HEATLEY, N. G. AND FLOREY, H. W., Brit. J. Pharmacol., 8 (1953) 252.
[8] ABRAHAM, E. P. AND NEWTON, G. C. F., Biochem. J., 58 (1954) 103.
[9] TOSONI, A. L., GLASS, D. G. AND GOLDSMITH, L., Biochem. J., 69 (1958) 476.
[10] BALLIO, A., CHAIN, E. B., DENTICE DI ACCADIO, F., BATCHELOR, F. R. AND ROLINSON, G. N., Nature, 183 (1959) 180.
[11] BATCHELOR, F. R., DOYLE, F. P., NAYLER, J. H. C. AND ROLINSON, G. N., Nature, 183 (1959) 257.
[12] ROLINSON, G. N. AND STEVENS, SHIRLEY, Proc. Roy. Soc. B, 154 (1961) 509.
[13] BATCHELOR, F.R., CHAIN, E.B. AND ROLINSON, G. N., Proc. Roy. Soc. B. 154 (1961) 478.

14 BATCHELOR, F. R., COLE, M., GAZZARD, D. AND ROLINSON, G. N., *Nature, 195* (1962) 954.
15 GRANT, N. H., CLARK, D. E. AND ALBURN, H. R., *J. Amer. chem. Soc., 84* (1962) 876.
16 GOUREVITCH, A., HUNT, G. A., LUTTINGER, J. R., CARMACK, C. C. AND LEIN, J., *Proc. Soc. exp. Biol. (N.Y.), 107* (1961) 455.
17 BRAIN, E. G., DOYLE, F. P., HARDY, K., LONG, A. A. W., MEHTA, M. D., MILLER, D., NAYLER, J. H. C., SOULAL, M. J., STOVE, E. R. AND THOMAS, G. R., *J. chem. Soc.,* (1962) 1445.
18 DOYLE, F. P., HARDY, K., NAYLER, J. H. C., SOULAL, M. J., STOVE E. R. AND WADDINGTON, H. R. J., *J. chem. Soc.,* (1962) 1453.
19 GOUREVITCH, A., HUNT, G. A. AND LEIN, J., *Antibiot. and Chemother., 10* (1960) 121.
20 PERRON, Y. G., MINOR, W. F., CRAST, L. B., GOUREVITCH, A., LEIN, J. AND CHENEY, L. C., *J. med. pharm. Chem., 5* (1962) 1016.
21 BRAIN, E. G., DOYLE, F. P., MEHTA, M. D., MILLER, D., NAYLER, J. H. C. AND STOVE, E. R., *J. chem. Soc.,* (1963) 491.
22 ROSENMAN, S. B. AND WARREN, G. H., *Antimicrobial Agents and Chemotherapy,* (1962) 369.
23 WHITEHOUSE, A. C., MORGAN, J. G., SCHUMACHER, JANET AND HAMBURGER, M., *Antimicrobial Agents and Chemotherapy,* (1962) 384.
24 RICHARDS, H. C., HOUSLEY, J. R. AND SPOONER, D. F., *Nature, 199* (1963) 354.
25 HESELTINE, W. W. AND FREEMAN, F. M., *J. Pharm. Pharmacol., 11,* (1960) 169.
26 DOYLE, F. P., NAYLER, J. H. C., WADDINGTON, H. R. J., HANSON, J. C. AND THOMAS, G. R., *J. chem. Soc.,* (1963) 497.
27 DOYLE, F. P., LONG, A. A. W., NAYLER, J. H. C. AND STOVE, E. R., *Nature 192* (1961) 1183.
28 NAYLER, J. H. C., LONG, A. A. W., BROWN, D. M., ACRED, P., ROLINSON, G. N., BATCHELOR, F. R., STEVENS, SHIRLEY AND SUTHERLAND, R. *Nature, 195* (1962) 1264.
29 SETO, T. A., HUANG, H. T., WEAVER, J. M., McBRIDE, J. T., ENGLISH, A. R. AND SHULL, G. M., *Proceedings of the Conference on Antimicrobial Agents, Washington, October 26–28,* Plenum Press, New York, 1960.
30 PERRON, Y. G., MINOR, W. F., CRAST, L. G. AND CHENEY, L. C., *J. org. Chem.,* (1961) 3365.
31 GOUREVITCH, A., HOLDREGE, C. T., HUNT, G. A., MINOR, W. F., FLANIGAN, C. C., CHENEY, L. C. AND LEIN, J., *Antibiot. Chemother., 12* (1962) 318.
32 NEWTON, G. G. F. AND ABRAHAM, E. P., *Biochem. J., 58* (1954) 103.
33 ROLINSON, G. N. AND STEVENS, SHIRLEY, *Brit. med. J., II* (1961) 191.
34 STEWART, G. T., COLES, H. M. T., NIXON, H. H. AND HOLT, R. J., *Brit. med. J., II* (1961) 200.
35 STEWART, G. T., *Pharmakotherapia, 1* (1963) 197.
36 DOYLE, F. P., FOSKER, G. R., NAYLER, J. H. C. AND SMITH, H., *J. chem. Soc.,* (1962) 1440.
37 TURNER, T. D. AND RUSSELL, A. D., *J. Pharm. Pharmacol., 14* (1962) 395.
38 GOUREVITCH, A., WOLFE, S. AND LEIN, J., *Antimicrobial Agents and Chemotherapy,* (1961) 576.
39 KNOX, R., *Nature, 192* (1961) 492.
40 BERRYMAN, G. H. AND SYLVESTER, J. C., *Antibiot. Ann.,* (1959–60) (1954) 521.
41 BOMAN, H. G. AND ERIKSSON, K. G., *J. gen. Microbiol., 31* (1963) 339.
42 FLOREY, H. W., CHAIN, E., HEATLEY, N. G., JENNINGS, M. A., SANDERS, A. G., ABRAHAM, E. P. AND FLOREY, M. E. (Eds.), *"Antibiotics",* Oxford University Press, 1949, p. 1097.
43 HOLT, R. J. AND STEWART, G. T., *J. gen. Microbiol., 36* (1964) 203.
44 HERR, E. B., *Antimicrobial Agents and Chemotherapy,* (1962) 201.

Chapter 11

THE MODE OF ACTION OF PENICILLINS. III

INTERACTIONS; CONCLUSIONS

INTERACTIONS WITH OTHER DRUGS

When penicillin first became available for therapy, the only other antibacterial drugs of any value were the sulphonamides and arsenicals. It was natural therefore that these substances should be tested in combination with penicillin to see if a better antibacterial effect could be obtained. The first recorded investigation is that of Ungar[1] who reported that sulphapyridine in sub-threshold doses increased the inhibitory action of penicillin against streptococci and staphylococci at least two-fold. This finding was confirmed with other sulphonamides[2–4] and other organisms, including *Brucella*[5]. It appeared at first that small amounts of sulphonamides potentiated the action of penicillin but, against some organisms, subinhibitory concentrations of penicillin increased the effect of sulphonamides[2]. Some inconsistencies were also apparent. Garrod[6] found that sulphathiazole reduced the bactericidal action of penicillin against staphylococci where Bigger[7] found that the same drug increased the bactericidal action on *S. typhi*. The phenomena of synergy, additive action and antagonism had not been closely studied before. Hobby and Dawson[8] showed that the effect of a given combination *in vitro* depended upon at least five variables—the concentration of each drug; inoculum; condition of growth; intrinsic sensitivity of organism to each individual drug; and species of organism.

The importance of these factors was agreed by other workers[9,10] and it soon became obvious—though the lesson has often been forgotten—that the conditions favouring synergy of action were so variable, even *in vitro*, that the chance of improving the action of penicillin by combining it with another drug were remote. Some combinations were antagonistic: helvolic acid, itself bactericidal to staphylococci, shielded the same organisms against the stronger bactericidal action of penicillin if added within five minutes[11]. Much later, the same kind of interference was found with chloramphenicol and tetracyclines[12]. The action of penicillin upon pyogenic cocci was so strong that no therapeutic advantage, and no obvious clue to its mode of action, seemed to emanate from its combination with other antibacterial agents[13]. The apparent synergy against *S. typhi*[7] suggested that combined therapy might be effective against relatively resistant gram-negative bacilli but closer investigation[14] threw doubt upon this idea. There was evidence that penicillin damaged resistant bacteria and thereby rendered them more susceptible to sulphonamides[15] but this kind of interaction can be obtained only under ideal conditions *in vitro* and there is no evidence that it is predictable or beneficial clinically. Data about combinations of the new penicillins with penicillin G, with each other, or with different drugs, is scanty but, again, there is no evidence of any significant enhancement of activity.

On theoretical grounds, there are good reasons for believing that bacteriostatic agents cannot enhance the action of a penicillin which is directed primarily against dividing cells. The addition of other bactericidal agents however seemed to offer no improvement. The only useful kind of synergy with a bactericidal drug is a combination which converts a partial bactericidal effect into a total one; this may occur if penicillin G and streptomycin act together upon *Streptococcus faecalis*[16] but is otherwise extremely rare. Himmelweit[17] found that phages accelerated the lysis of staphylococci by penicillin. When confirmed later[18] it was noted that this occurred without any antecedent swelling or other morphological change, as assessed by ultraviolet and electron microscopy.

INTERACTIONS WITH SUBSTANCES OTHER THAN DRUGS

In addition to drugs, many other substances are known to potentiate or interfere with the action of penicillin *in vitro*. Triphenylmethane dyes, among others, are often powerfully bactericidal to vegetative bacterial cells, and some of these potentiate the action of penicillin. In a review of the problem, Pratt and Dufrenoy[19] formed the opinion that dyes acted as hydrogen acceptors, favouring the conversion SH → SS. Interference with sulphydryl groups was also suggested by these investigators as an explanation of the potentiating effect of cobalt and bismuth ions. They reasoned that the dehydrogenation of sulphydryl groups caused at first an increase in metabolism then a failure of respiratory enzymes to provide enough energy for concentrating extracellular substances in the vacuoles. The SH ⇌ SS equilibrium shifted to the right leading to a rise in oxidation–reduction potential which killed the cell. Arsenicals, notably phenyl arsenoxides, are known to enhance the action of penicillin upon spirochaetes very strongly, *in vitro* and *in vivo*; Eagle and his colleagues[20,21] suggested that blockage of essential SH groups was involved in this interaction also. Detergents and phages accelerated lysis by exposing sulphydryl groups to dehydrogenation but cysteine antagonised the lytic action of penicillin by donating extra sulphydryl groups. Florey and his colleagues had pointed out that any thiol should do this, which was not the case. It had been suggested earlier that the amino group of cysteine react-ed with penicillin to form a penicilloic acid peptide[22]. Other amino acids also antagonised the action of penicillin[23]. These included the dicarboxy-monoamino acids (*e.g.* glutamic) together with cystine, arginine, histidine and hydroxyproline. The action on gram-negative bacilli was said to be antagonised more strongly than that on gram-positive organisms but it is not clear how, if at all, this antagonism relates to the effect of penicillin, studied by Gale and his colleagues (Chapter 9) on amino acid assimilation. What-ever the explanation of these happenings, it is clear that the action of peni-cillin in any environment is profoundly influenced by a variety of other sub-stances and that any study, especially biochemical study, of the mode of action has to take these variables into account. In the light of subsequent knowledge, the dehydrogenation of sulphydryl groups, the consequent rise in oxidation–reduction potential, the loss of the gram reaction[24] are non-specific changes, the results and not the primary cause of damage to the bacterial cell.

GENERAL CONCLUSIONS

Facts, as food for thought, have to be assimilated before they can be digested. Few of the investigators who have reported the mode of action of penicillin have been in possession of all the relevant facts even at the time of writing. The earlier workers observed the physical changes in penicillin-treated or-ganisms without any clue as to their biochemical basis. The first biochemical studies were conducted at high concentrations, without reference to the physical effects which were known to occur, often optimally, at much lower concentrations. Many results have been reported, and hypotheses elaborat-ed, upon single species of organisms without recognition of intra-species variation in sensitivity to penicillin. The main pathways of investigation to date of the effects of penicillin can be summarised as follows:

Morphological and physical effects
(*a*) Swelling of the cell and inhibition of its division
(*b*) Induction of spheroblasts, protoplasts and L-forms
(*c*) Binding to a specific component in the cell

Biochemical effects
(*a*) Accumulation of nucleotide precursors of cell-wall material
(*b*) Inhibition of mucopeptide synthesis
(*c*) Potentiation by dehydrogenation of SH groups
(*d*) Inhibition of incorporation of amino acids
(*e*) Inhibition of enzyme synthesis (sometimes offset by induction of penicillinase-formation)

Structure–activity relationships
(*a*) Influence of side-chain
(*b*) Steric considerations
(*c*) Influence of basic group

In the writer's opinion, it is at present impossible to fuse these diverse leads into a working hypothesis, unless it be for the purpose of evoking further "healthy scepticism"[25] preferably based upon plain rather than upon ornate facts. Nevertheless, some of these approaches are converging and it is important to see where they lead.

The main advance is undoubtedly the characterisation of what is now usually referred to as a specific "biochemical lesion". This is the inhibition of formation of mucopeptide which is the most important component conferring rigidity upon the cell wall, certainly of staphylococci, probably of some other gram-positive cocci and possibly of some gram-negative bacilli. It is a reasonable assumption that, deprived of this rigid support, the limiting cytoplasmic membrane yields to the internal osmotic pressure of the cell contents, causing lysis and death of the cell. Growing as they do under conditions of high osmolarity, which safeguards them from this danger, L-forms of staphylococci are highly resistant to penicillin. This much is known, with fair certainty, about penicillin G and staphylococci; the same probably applies to methicillin, quinacillin[26] and staphylococci; there is some evidence that certain streptococci are similarly affected by penicillin G. Detailed references in support of these conclusions are quoted in the foregoing text. But there the factual information ends. Even with staphylococci, the rest is conjecture, for there are no detailed reports available concerning the binding of newer penicillins, the accumulation within the treated cell of nucleotide precursors of muramic and teichoic acids or of the response of resistant strains, excepting the limited experiments of Rogers and his colleagues[27] with methicillin. The only certain information concerning other gram-positive cocci is their susceptibility to lysis, and some other similarities in pattern of response to the penicillins; but susceptibility varies greatly, many strains of streptococci being naturally resistant to conventional concentrations of several penicillins. With gram-negative bacilli, the position is even less complete. Substances specific to mucopeptides, including 2,6-diaminopimelic acid[28] as well as muramic acid, D-alanine and D-glutamic acid, are present in the cell wall but in low concentrations[29]. It is therefore questionable whether interference with the synthesis of mucopeptide, which probably amounts to less than 5% of cell-wall substance[25], can by itself damage the cell sufficiently or whether, for that matter, mucopeptide is responsible for the rigidity of the cell wall. This difference in gram-negative bacilli might seem to explain their relative resistance to penicillin, for it is a fact that both penicillin G and ampicillin cause 50% inhibition of mucopeptide synthesis[30] in *Esch. coli*, but it does not explain the much higher susceptibility of gram-negative organisms in general, or of enterococci, to ampicillin. Again, if the penicillin-binding theory applies, the amount bound per unit of membrane in a bacillus, which elongates as it divides, might well be absolutely or relatively insufficient to inhibit mucopeptide formation. In an admittedly speculative comment on this question, Rogers[25] suggests that the double-thickness membrane at the annulus might bind more penicillin, leading to a local inhibition of mucopeptide formation and hence of cell division. This explanation would accord with morphological observations[31,32] and, if only a few relatively sensitive strains of *Esch. coli*, *Proteus* or *Salmonella* are examined, seems plausible; if a more representative collection is considered, the intra-species variation would seem to exclude such an explanation. However, the fact, first stated by Duguid in 1946, that virtually all species are to some extent affected by penicillin, shows that a fundamental metabolic process is affected, for it is, equally, an unassailable fact that the action of penicillin is indirect. The ready induction of spheroblasts shows also that the main interference is with division rather than enlargement; there is no evidence that synthesis of protein or nucleic acid is primarily affected.

The difference in susceptibility between species is therefore not completely explained by any known differences in cell-structure or composition, while the variation within species has hardly been explored in this way. This is where considerations of structure in relation to activity are more informative, and perhaps more useful. The addition of a free basic group (NH$_2$) undoubtedly confers wider activity upon the penicillin molecule while, conversely lengthening or hindering of the side-chain narrows the spectrum. Those correlations are probably as definite as any, and much more so than most, in this perplexing field. A site of activity can therefore be located in and around the side-chain. There is a gap in knowledge concerning the role of penicillins with modified side-chains and basic groups in the metabolism of sensitive and resistant organisms. If this gap is to be filled, the newer penicillins must now be used systematically as research tools but they must be tested against sensitive and resistant bacteria, between and within species. Until this has been done, our knowledge of the mode of action of penicillins is incomplete, perhaps dangerously so. Had it not been for the advent of the newer penicillins, the mucopeptide story might have seemed adequate as an explanation of the mode of action of "penicillin" and, even now[25], it is difficult to avoid viewing it with "peculiar satisfaction". It is to be hoped also that the proponents and extrapolators of bacterial chemistry will one day confound the empiricists with a successful therapeutic prediction. To quote the words of Rogers[25]: ". . . in few fields have theoretical studies paid such poor dividends and the empirical approach been so triumphant as in the study of antibiotics". This would still be a true if gloomy ending to the chapter, but there is comfort in the reflection that the empiricists are still at work, synthesising as well as analysing.

REFERENCES

[1] UNGAR, J., Nature, 152 (1943) 245.
[2] RAMMELKAMP, C. H. AND KEEFER, C. S., J. clin. Invest., 22 (1943) 649.
[3] BIGGER, J. W., Lancet, ii (1944) 142.
[4] KIRBY, W. M. M., Proc. Soc. exp. Biol. (N.Y.), 57 (1944) 149.
[5] T'UNG, T., Proc. Soc. exp. Biol. (N.Y.), 66 (1944) 8.
[6] GARROD, L. P., Lancet, ii (1944) 673.
[7] BIGGER, J. W., Lancet, i (1946) 81.
[8] HOBBY, G. L. AND DAWSON, M. H., J. Bact., 51 (1946) 447.
[9] KLEIN, M. AND KALTER, S. S., J. Bact., 51 (1946) 95.
[10] KLEIN, M. AND KIMMELMAN, L. J., J. Bact., 52 (1946) 471.
[11] CHAIN, E. AND DUTHIE, E. S., Lancet, i (1945) 562.
[12] JAWETZ, E. AND GUNNISON, J. B., Antibiot. and Chemotherapy, 2 (1952) 243.
[13] KLEIN, M. AND KIMMELMAN, L. J., J. Bact., 64 (1947) 363.
[14] THOMAS, J. C. AND HAYES, W., J. Hyg. (Camb.), 45 (1947) 313.
[15] STEWART, G. T., J. Hyg. (Camb), 45 (1947) 282.
[16] BARBER, MARY AND GARROD, L. P., Antibiotics and Chemotherapy. Livingstone, Edinburgh, London, 1963.
[17] HIMMELWEIT, F., Lancet, ii (1945) 104.
[18] SMILES, J., WELCH, F. V. AND ELFORD, W. J., J. gen. Microbiol., 2 (1948) 220.
[19] PRATT, R. AND DUFRENOY, J., Bact. Rev., 12 (1948) 79.

[20] EAGLE, H., MAGNUSON, H. J. AND FLEISCHMAN, R., *J. vener. Dis. Inform.*, *27* (1946) 3.
[21] EAGLE, H. AND MUSSALMAN, A. D., *J. exp. Med.*, *88* (1948) 99.
[22] Squibb Institute for Medical Research, *Report No. 34*, Nov. 1944.
[23] SCHWARZMAN, G., *J. exp. Med.*, *83* (1946) 65.
[24] HENRY, H. AND STACEY, B., *Proc. roy. Soc. B.*, *133* (1946) 391.
[25] ROGERS, H. J., In *Resistance of bacteria to the penicillins*, Ciba Foundation Study Group No. 13, Churchill, London, 1962.
[26] HUGO, W. B. AND STRETTON, R. G., *Nature*, *202* (1964) 1217.
[27] ROGERS, H. J. AND JELJASZEWICZ, J., *Biochem. J.*, *81* (1961) 576.
[28] SALTON, M. R. J., *Nature*, *180* (1957) 338.
[29] MANDELSTAM, J., *Biochem. J.*, *84* (1962) 294.
[30] ROGERS, H. J. AND MANDELSTAM, J., *Biochem. J.*, *84* (1962) 299.
[31] FLEMING, A. VOUREKA, A., KRAMER, I. R. H. AND HUGHES, W. H. H., *J. gen. Microbiol.*, *4* (1950) 257.
[32] MURRAY, R. G. E., FRANCOMBE, W. H. AND MAYALL, B. H., *Canad. J. Microbiol.*, *5* (1959) 641.

Chapter 12

TOXICITY AND PHARMACOLOGY

More so even than its selective antibacterial action, the inimitable quality of penicillin is its lack of toxicity. This was noted by Fleming in tests with the crude brew, which could be given to rabbits intravenously and could be added to suspensions of human leucocytes without detriment[1]. Later, when successive batches were being purified, Welch and his colleagues[2] found that the toxicity of the sodium salt to mice was very close to that of sodium acetate— in other words, such toxicity as there was could be attributed to the sodium cation; if a more toxic cation is substituted (lithium, ammonium, strontium, calcium, magnesium, potassium, in that order) the toxicity rises. Potassium is the most toxic cation, though the potassium salts, being highly soluble, are often used in therapeutic preparations, especially of the α-phenoxymethyl penicillins (see p. 30) as well as in certain preparations of penicillin G.

Toxicity can also occur at therapeutic dosage with complex formulations designed to secure long-action or selective localisation. Apart from this, 6-APA and its main biosynthetic derivatives appear to be almost as free from direct toxicity as penicillin G itself. The main hazard with all the penicillins is indirect toxicity arising usually from hypersensitivity or from suppression of the competitive bacterial flora in the orifices and gut during therapy.

RESULTS IN ANIMALS

It was established by 1945 that most laboratory animals tolerated penicillin G in large doses, given for weeks on end orally or parenterally. In mice and rats, the LD_{50} is of the order of 2 g/kg or more, on continued administration and, even then, death is probably due to the cation and volume of injection. Other species, including dogs, cats and monkeys, have also received large doses (0.25–0.5 g/kg) repeatedly for pharmacological tests without suffering, while the widespread use of penicillin in veterinary practice has extended testing to almost every domestic and farmyard animal; even fish and plants have been reared in water containing penicillin. The newer penicillins have been less intensively examined but enough data is available (Table XI) to indicate that, in their lack of immediate toxicity, they are comparable to penicillin G.

TABLE XI

TOLERANCE OF VARIOUS SPECIES TO PENICILLINS

Drug	Dose tolerated (mg/kg/day) parenterally						Acute LD_{50}* (mice or rats)
	Mouse	Rat	Guinea-pig	Rabbit	Dog	Man	
Penicillin G	3000	3500	5	500	500	1000	> 5000
Methicillin	3000	4000	10	500	250	400	5000
Ampicillin	2000	5000				150	> 5000
Cloxacillin	2000	500	10	200		100	> 4000

* Limited by solubility and volume of injection.

The best-known exception to this general rule is the guinea pig. At an early stage[3] it was noted that some guinea pigs died 2–3 days after injections of 2000 units of impure penicillins; removal of impurities did not lessen this toxicity[4] for it was found that deaths occurred with doses as low as 7–12 mg penicillin G, though some guinea pigs tolerated larger doses and could receive enough to be cured of experimental leptospirosis[5]. Guinea pigs are susceptible also to the newer penicillins which can be lethal in doses of 10–20 mg.

The reason for this high susceptibility of the guinea pig is incompletely understood. There are no consistent organic changes post-mortem except for generalised vasodilatation and distension of the gut. Pulmonary congestion, adrenal necrosis, interference with vitamin metabolism and necrosis of cardiac muscle[3] have also been suggested as mechanisms. The only other animal known to have similar susceptibility is the Syrian hamster, which may die on the 3rd, 4th or 5th day after a single dose given subcutaneously or intra-peritoneally[6]. Death is preceded by signs of vasodilatation and shock. It is known that the intestinal flora of these rodents consist largely of lactobacilli and other gram-positive organisms which are sensitive to the action of penicillin and it is possible therefore that the apparent toxicity of the penicillins in some of these animals is due to suppression of the predominant gram-positive flora with release of, or superinfection by, coliform bacilli to which the guinea pig is known to be vulnerable. The post-mortem findings are consistent with this explanation, as is the fact that deaths do not occur before the 3rd day. This suggests that toxicity in the guinea-pig is a secondary or indirect process. The acute LD_{50} of single oral doses is about 5 g/kg[7] compared with 8 g/kg in mice, whereas the chronic LD_{50} is of the order of 0.3 g/kg as against 4 g/kg in mice. Acute toxicity in any species is shown by convulsions and respiratory failure, with gastro-intestinal irritation if the drug is given orally; these effects are probably attributable to the cation, for large doses of the free acid are well tolerated when given by mouth. Chronic toxicity in any species produces distension of the gut, especially the caecum, which may be hypertrophied. Cats, dogs, rats and mice withstand these effects for months on end but guinea pigs succumb in 3–10 days*. Culture filtrates of the secondary coliform flora[8] cause similar deaths with prostration, hypothermia and respiratory failure. According to Carlson and Walker[9], the toxic agent is the lipopolysaccharide endotoxin of *Esch. coli*, which replaces the penicillin-sensitive lactobacillary flora; this toxin is demonstrable by the fluorescent-antibody technique in the kidney, liver and spleen, which may therefore explain the sudden vasodilatation and shock which suddenly occur in these animals.

These animal studies demonstrate the importance, with any antibacterial drug given orally, of drawing a distinction between primary or intrinsic toxicity due to the action of the drug upon the recipient's tissues, and secondary or indirect toxicity due to changes in the bacterial flora of the gut. This difference, which is seldom appreciated in conventional toxicology, is in turn dependent upon environmental factors such as the air-borne flora, atmospheric humidity, cross-infection, feeding habits and so forth. These factors are collectively almost impossible to control but they obviously have considerable bearing upon secondary toxicity arising in the course of therapeutic dosage in medical and veterinary practice.

RESULTS IN MAN

Penicillin G is the yardstick against which any new penicillin must be compared; but the upper limit of safe dosage of penicillin G in man has never been determined. By 1946 it was established that intravenous doses of 10 mega units daily could be tolerated almost indefinitely in the treatment of

---

* Recent studies by Steinman *et al.* (J. Bact., *88* (1964) 537) indicate that penicillin G is non-toxic to guinea pigs delivered by caesarean section and reared under "germ-free" conditions.

bacterial endocarditis[10]. Since then, record dosages have been achieved and surpassed by successive investigators, without adverse reactions. One of the latest and most convincing instances of the lack of intrinsic toxicity of penicillin G was the case of clostridial infection and *Esch. coli* septicaemia treated by Bigby and Jones[11]. This patient received 17 mega units in six days, during which she was almost anuric and had a blood urea of 360–550 mg%; both infections were cured. In recent years, Spitzy[12] of Vienna has used enormous doses of penicillin G, orally and parenterally, in the treatment of a variety of acute and chronic infections, including several for which penicillin is not usually considered eligible. Apart from their therapeutic interest, Spitzy's studies have shown that doses of 120 mega units per day are well-tolerated.

The use of such large doses of penicillin G was justified by necessity in the early days when no satisfactory alternatives were available for the treatment of severe infections or relatively resistant organisms. Since no comparable necessity now exists, it is unlikely that the newer penicillins will be pushed to the same levels; nevertheless, doses which would be large by any other standard have already been given (Table XII), without incident. Methicillin has been given intravenously to patients with staphylococcal endocarditis in doses of over 20 g per day[13,14]; newborn babies with infected Spitz–Holter valves and septicaemia have received total doses of over 100 g[15] without

TABLE XII

USE OF LARGE DOSES OF THE NEWER PENICILLINS

Drug	Duration (weeks)	Daily (g)	Total (g)	Route	Conditions	Reference
ethicillin	"Several"	24	>600	IV	Endocarditis	13
ethicillin	11	200 mg/kg	104	IM and IV	Septicaemia (infants)	15
ethicillin		4–20	270	IV	Septicaemia	59
ethicillin	not stated	20	—	IV	Various staphylococcal infections	14
npicillin	12	50–100 mg/kg	168	IM and IV	Endocarditis	16
npicillin	not stated	4	not stated	IM and IV	Various	60
npicillin		150 mg/kg	not stated	IM and IV	Meningitis (children)	17
npicillin	not stated	385 mg/kg	not stated	oral	Various	61
npicillin	12	3–4	260	oral	Typhoid carriers	62
acillin	6	50–100	—	IM and IV	Staphylococcal infections	63

References p. 138/139

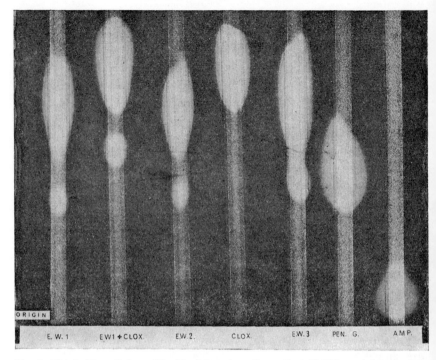

Fig. 8. Metabolites of cloxacillin (clox) in urine of a patient (E.W.) receiving the drug orally. Penicillin G and ampicillin (amp) are shown for comparison. Chromatographic bio-assay.

evidence of immediate or delayed toxicity. Ampicillin has been used in doses of 4 g/day in the treatment of endocarditis due to *Str. faecalis*[16] and can be given safely to children with meningitis in intermittent or continuous intravenous dosage at the rate of 100–200 mg/kg/day[17]. Penicillin V and phenethicillin are well tolerated orally in doses of 8 g/day[18]. The isoxazoles oxacillin and cloxacillin have been used by various workers in doses up to 6 g/day, orally or parenterally, but there is no record to date of sustained higher dosage with these drugs or with other derivatives of 6-APA such as nafcillin, phenbenicillin or propicillin; except for mild gastro-intestinal disturbances, all of these drugs appear to be devoid of immediate toxicity within the therapeutic range (20–80 mg/kg/day).

From these results, it is not too early to say that the newer penicillins at present in therapeutic use resemble penicillin G in that they lack direct toxicity; methicillin and ampicillin are clearly safe in doses well above the standard. It is impossible however to be sure that any of the newer derivatives are as innocuous as penicillin G; even if equally large doses (1–2 g/kg/day) were given—and it is difficult to foresee any need for this, except possibly with ampicillin—some time would have to elapse before delayed toxicity could be excluded. It is already known (see Chapter 14) that all the main derivatives of 6-APA are cross-allergenic and, in view of the diversity of penicillin allergy, it is possible that some derivatives may provoke organic reactions more easily than penicillin G does; the examples of idiosyncrasy attributed to methicillin (see below) may come into this category. There is evidence also that phenethicillin and the isoxazoles (Fig 8) are subjected to a greater degree of metabolic conversion than penicillin G, methicillin or ampicillin, and this also could be a factor conducive to toxicity if large doses are given. Before considering further the question of potential toxicity, it is instructive to consider the reasons why the unmodified penicillin molecule is non-toxic.

REASONS FOR THE NON-TOXICITY OF PENICILLINS

6-APA is a simple molecule, composed of two cyclically-fused amino acids, L-valine and L-cysteine (p. 18). All the existing therapeutic derivatives are simple acyl dipeptides. The principal side-chains, such a phenylacetic acid, dimethoxybenzoic acid and the α-phenoxyalkyls, are in themselves no more toxic than the dipeptide. Provided that the side-chains do not become unduly complex or toxic in their own right, the penicillins are unlikely to become unreceptive physiologically.

Despite its simple structure, the penicillin molecule is selectively toxic to nearly all bacterial cells, though in varying degree. The work of Park and others (Chapter 9) has shown that this is mainly due to inhibition of mucopeptide synthesis in the cell wall. The biochemical pathways of this synthesis, muramic and teichoic acids, are not represented in mammalian cells which are therefore indifferent to the presence of penicillins, even in high concentration. This is well shown by the extraordinary tolerance of various mammalian cells of human or animal origin growing in tissue-culture to constant high concentrations of most—though not all—penicillins (Table XIII). By reason of its differential action, penicillin is nowadays an invariable constituent of most tissue-culture media.

The penicillins are to some extent metabolised by animal cells but the metabolites so far identified are not known to be directly toxic. Some metabolites, like penicillenic acid and penicilloyl moieties, can be indirectly toxic

TABLE XIII

EFFECT OF PENICILLINS UPON CELLS GROWING IN TISSUE-CULTURE

Penicillin (µg/ml)	HeLa	Effect on Monkey kidney	Embryo kidney
Penicillin G 1000	No interference with growth or morphology in 4 days		
Methicillin 1000	*do.*		
Ampicillin 1000	No abnormality	Growth ceased at 3rd day	No abnormality
Ampicillin 100	No interference with growth or morphology in 4 days		
Cloxacillin 1000	Toxic changes 1st day irreversible	Reversible toxic changes	Minor morphological changes
Cloxacillin 100	Growth ceased on 3rd day	Reversible toxic changes	Minor morphological changes
Isoxazole 1702, 1000	Death on 3rd day		Irreversible toxic changes, 4th day
Isoxazole 1702, 100	Reversible toxic changes		

by conjugating with proteins to act as sensitising antigens (Chapter 14); this may happen as a result of degradation outside or inside the body. Other metabolites, such as those formed from the α-phenoxy derivatives and the isoxazoles, are probably the result of relatively simple metabolic conversions in hepatic or other cells; these are discussed in detail later in this chapter but it can be said here that none has yet been shown to be toxic, though the process of metabolic conversion deserves much further attention.

The final major factor ensuring non-toxicity is the rapid excretion of the penicillins. At an early stage the Oxford workers[19] found that penicillin recovered from the urine was freed from pyrogenic impurity by passage through the body. Since then, it has been repeatedly shown that penicillin G is rapidly excreted by the normal kidney in strict proportion to the amount injected and the circulating plasma concentration[20]. Elimination is due to glomerular clearance and tubular excretion and, if renal function is normal, usually accounts for 73–99% of an injected dose within 6 h[21]. Other penicillins are excreted similarly but not identically. The renal clearance of penicillins G, X and F is the same as the calculated renal plasma flow[22] and, therefore, the glomerular filtration rate. This is independent, within wide limits, of the concentration of penicillin in the plasma, though, if very large doses are given, tubular excretion rises sharply and is probably responsible for the rapid fall in high plasma concentrations. Penicillin K is cleared at only half the rate, with a relatively higher glomerular clearance. This may be due in part to greater protein binding which affects also some of the newer derivatives such as the α-phenoxy and isoxazole derivatives which are not excreted in the urine so freely as penicillin G or methicillin[23]. Blockage of tubular excretion by carinamide[24] or probenecid[25] permits blood and tissue levels to be raised and sustained without toxicity. Even in patients with diminished renal function amounting to anuria or oliguria, some of the penicillins are well-tolerated. Of the newer penicillins, all except the isoxazoles are excreted by glomerules and tubules[26].

Apart from rapid renal excretion, biliary excretion is also known to be a significant factor affecting the new as well as the older penicillins[27,28]. As in the urine, the drugs are largely unchanged in the bile, though metabolites of the isoxazoles can be detected. This means that both real and hepatic excretion proceed without the subtraction of energy from the cells that would result if, like many other drugs, the penicillins had to be metabolised before excretion. In consequence, no matter how great the load, the liver and kidneys do not show toxic change structurally or functionally when penicillins are administered. This happy position will of course depend upon the continuing non-toxicity of the side-chains; with the isoxazole derivatives there is an indication from tissue-culture studies (Table XIII) and metabolism (p. 41) that chemical limitations are in sight.

The fraction of a penicillin which is not excreted appears to be inactivated. Even outside the body, most penicillins undergo some degradation in solution at 37° to penicillenic acid and other inactive products. In the presence of serum and various tissues, this process is accelerated[29]. Part of the loss probably occurs in the gut after biliary excretion[27] and it is possible that intestinal bacteria play a part in this. Traces of penicillins can be detected in tears, mucin and breast milk but little or none in sweat or faeces. The bulk of a given dose is therefore accounted for by renal excretion, mainly of unchanged drug, partly of metabolites; a smaller fraction by biliary excretion; and the remainder—usually less than 10%—by inactivation within the body.

From the above data, it is obvious that the 6-APA molecule and its simple derivatives are devoid of intrinsic toxicity to mammalian cells. Penicillin G can circulate harmlessly in the body in concentrations of about 50 mg% which means that it is less toxic than many of the body's own metabolites and crystalloids, and probably no more toxic than simple amino acids, glucose or urea. Its excretion pattern is direct and rapid. There is evidence that the newer penicillins are also accepted by the body in the same, virtually physiological, role though the effect of massive doses has not yet been assessed except in the case of methicillin. Since these considerations exclude direct toxicity, the penicillins must therefore be assessed in terms of their indirect toxicity which is by no means negligible.

INDIRECT TOXICITY

Cation

Potassium and calcium are the most toxic of the cations supplied by the therapeutic salts of the various penicillins. Calcium has not so far been used in the new series of penicillins. Potassium is still the selected salt in certain preparations of penicillin G, and in α-phenoxy derivatives, notably penicillin V and phenethicillin which are employed in large doses in the treatment of endocarditis[18]. One mega unit of the potassium salt of penicillin G supplies 1.6 mequiv. of K^+. If 15 mega units are being administered daily, especially if renal function is imperfect, the 25 mequiv. of K^+ which is being administered parenterally may be cumulatively toxic; such doses are usually given in endocarditis and the heart, already damaged, may become dilated as a result. Large doses of the α-phenoxy penicillins given orally are much less liable to cause this effect, since intestinal absorption of the cation is balanced by excretion; also, the doses so far employed (up to 8 g/day) would be incapable of causing potassium intoxication unless there was serious renal insufficiency or unless a tubular blocking agent was being given. In this event, the daily load would be 15 mequiv. or more. This is the only circumstance in which the sodium cation (in penicillin G, methicillin and the isoxazoles) could also be toxic.

Changes in the normal bacterial flora

Surprisingly enough, there is still no certainty about what constitutes a normal buccal or intestinal flora in man and animals. One reason for this is that the limits of normality are very wide, varying with age, climate, season, diet and numerous other factors. In man, the flora of the mouth and pharynx is predominantly coccal, comprising gram-positive species such as α- or non-haemolytic streptococci, micrococci and *Neisseriae*; apart from *Haemophilus*, gram-negative bacilli are scanty or absent, and the flora is sensitive to all the penicillins, those with the widest spectra (ampicillin and penicillin G) having the strongest inhibitory effect. During penicillin therapy, therefore, this sensitive oropharyngeal flora is suppressed or eliminated, to be replaced partly by coliforms, partly by resistant streptococci or *Neisseriae*. If therapy is intensive, this happens quickly: coliforms can usually be detected within a day or two and, within four days, there may be a complete replacement of sensitive streptococci by resistant ones[30]. Inhalation therapy promotes these changes very quickly but also limits re-colonisation by all except the most resistant species; oral therapy, especially with flavoured suspensions and syrups, also hastens the change in flora, but the same change soon occurs even if the penicillins are given as tablets, capsules or injections.

In adults eating a mixed diet, the flora of the small intestine is scanty, containing enterococci, *Bacteroides* and lactobacilli, but few coliforms; in the large intestine, *Esch. coli* and *Bacteroides* proliferate more rapidly, though many other organisms, including anaerobic species, are also present. The effects of penicillins upon this complex flora vary. Enterococci and various sensitive bacilli are partly or completely suppressed; *Esch. coli* is suppressed by ampicillin[31] but not by the other penicillins; resistant organisms like *A. aerogenes*, *Ps. pyocyanea* and some strains of *Proteus*, if present, are unaffected or may increase proportionately as the more sensitive competitive flora is suppressed. The effect of the penicillins upon the coliforms is determined also by whether or not the individual strains form the inactivating enzymes amidase or β-lactamase (Chapter 13). If these enzymes are formed, the changes are minimal. There is, in any event, a tendency for persistence or superinfection by coliforms which produce β-lactamase (p. 142) and these organisms may colonise the small intestine and oropharynx as well as the colon. Penicillin therapy may also inhibit the acidophilic Döderlein flora of the vagina. In many individuals, these changes in bacterial flora are symptomless, and are quickly readjusted when therapy ceases. Chemoprophylaxis with penicillin V (Chapter 4) has been conducted for long periods without difficulty. The normal bacterial flora is however defensive, if only in the competitive sense, toward extraneous infection. If penicillinase-forming organisms, especially staphylococci, are in the vicinity, superinfection is liable to occur. Until the advent of the penicillinase-resistant penicillins, this was the greatest hazard of institutional therapy with penicillins G or V. Secondary pharyngeal colonisation by coliforms is seldom a cause of trouble except in infants, or in patients with chronic respiratory disease, debility (malnutrition, malignancy) or weakened defences (leukaemia, steroids, renal disease). Changes in the coliform balance of the gut are usually symptomless but may be associated with diarrhoea, malabsorption and pruritis ani. The presence of amidase-forming or β-lactamase-forming coliforms high in the small gut might conceivably lead to inactivation of certain penicillins given orally. In practice, this seems to be unimportant. The excretion of 6-APA in urine has been reported[32] presumably as a consequence of deacylation of penicillin V in the gut. The writer has been unable to find this metabolite in patients and volunteers receiving penicillin V, not even when an amidase-forming coliform was given simultaneously in a capsule, and shown to have colonised the gut. It is probable that coliforms are unable to multiply sufficiently in the adverse conditions of the absorptive area of the small gut to have any effect upon the large quantity of penicillin present. Other metabolites of penicillins have not been identified in human faeces but a metabolite of cloxacillin is formed in the intestine of the rat[26].

One of the most common forms of secondary colonisation is that due to various species of *Saccharomycetes*. These yeasts are often present normally in the mouth and intestine, and increase in numbers during any form of antibacterial therapy. The main pathogenic yeast, *Candida albicans*, may also by present in health. It has therefore been assumed that stomatitis and other forms of active monilial infection are provoked during antibiotic therapy by a lessening of the growth of pharyngeal or intestinal bacteria, some of which are certainly inhibitory toward *C. albicans*, though others are neutral or even stimulatory. The outcome is determined by an interplay of metabolic factors arising from the growth of the various organisms[33] and changing the intra-intestinal environment. Restraint of *Candida* by bacterial growth may be due to simultaneous overgrowth of secondary bacterial invaders such as *Proteus*[34], themselves the result of antibiotic intervention, though there is no evidence that any intestinal bacteria are capable of producing antifungal substances[35]. If overgrowth of *Candida* occurs, the development of lesions is favoured by localising factors such as dentures, devitalised epithelium and bronchial disease[36]. Under these conditions, prolonged use of antibiotics undoubtedly provokes moniliasis[37]. Overgrowth of *Candida* in the gut can be prevented by the simultaneous administration of the polyene fungistatic agents[38] though this does not necessarily prevent colonisation of the respiratory tract.

The ecology of bacterial and fungal superinfection is therefore a problem of great complexity, and it is difficult to define measures which will ensure complete protection. It is important in the first place to look at the problem epidemiologically. If penicillinase-forming staphylococci are present, the likelihood of superinfection is high and a penicillinase-resistant penicillin should be employed where possible in preference to penicillin G or the phenoxymethyl penicillins. Staphylococal infection may in itself predispose to moniliasis[39] and, in the prolonged therapy necessary in staphylococcal endocarditis or fibrocystic disease, it is wise to anticipate this contingency by giving a polyene fungistatic agent earlier rather than later. In some situations, especially in warm climates, *Candida* is more common as a cause of stomatitis, oesophagitis, dermatitis and vaginitis, and may spread by cross-infection. In wounds and burns, secondary infection by *Ps. pyocyanea* and *Proteus* have long been recognised as the main risks of antibiotic therapy, and these organisms may also invade the urinary tract during instrumentation of patients treated with ampicillin[40].

Superinfection is less likely to arise with the penicillins than with tetracyclines but the risk is always present and each patient requires individual assessment. If prolonged or intensive therapy with penicillins is instituted, the pharyngeal and faecal flora should be sampled regularly. The presence of fungal hyphae in direct smears from the mouth or faeces, or of a newly-acquired *Staph. aureus*, give early warning of trouble, though lesser changes especially in the coliform flora can often be ignored. Where intensive antibacterial therapy is being practised, there is much to be said—microbiologically rather than psychologically—for the use of "pathogen-free patient-care areas" as described recently in Richmond, Virginia[41].

Hypersensitivity

This is undoubtedly the most common, the most difficult and the most dangerous side-effect in penicillin therapy. The new penicillins have increased rather than lessened this problem, for they are all cross- allergenic and cross-immunogenic with penicillin G and probably with each other (Chapter 14). Any therapeutic preparation of penicillin may act as a sensitising dose and it is possible that traces of penicillin in food, especially milk, may aggravate the development of the hypersensitive state. Sensitisation is most likely to be initiated by topical applications[42], especially in those who subsequently handle the drug; in such cases subsequent reactions may be characterised by pruritis and dermatitis at the original site of sensitisation, even when only a small test dose is given intradermally. Application to intact skin or mucous membranes is less likely to cause sensitisation than application to areas of eczema, burns or inflammation. Curiously enough, instillation of penicillin into abscess cavities or the subarachnoid space seems to be very rare as a cause of hypersensitivity. Parenteral administration is much more commonly associated with subsequent hypersensitivity than is oral administration. The use of depot preparations or long-acting derivatives[43] (*e.g.* benzathine or benethamine penicillin) increases the risk, both of initiating and of eliciting allergic reactions. Inhalation therapy with penicillin aerosols is known to carry some risk to asthmatics but there are few instances of reactions by this route in other patients.

Toxic reactions in sensitised subjects

The immuno-chemical mechanisms associated with hypersensitivity are extremely complex. There is good evidence that the most important antigenic determinant is a penicilloyl protein, formed usually by conjugation of penicillin or its degradation products by covalent bonding to tissue proteins. The penicillin is therefore a hapten and many of the signs of hypersensitivity follow the familiar pattern of delayed urticaria or serum sickness following second or subsequent injections of an unacceptable protein, with anaphylaxis in the most highly sensitised subjects. The basic lesion is urticaria, provoked by release of histamine or other irritants from the combination of antibody with antigen in the affected site or sites; this leads to a local increase in vascular permeability, oedema, pruritis and any or all of the features of inflammation. In the most simple instance, as in a scratch test, the reaction is confined to epidermal cells and dermal vessels, lymphatics and nerve-endings in a few millimeters of skin though, in highly-sensitised individuals, less than 1 μg of a penicillin or penicilloyl conjugate can evoke this reaction[44]. If a larger dose or larger volume of penicillin is given, this reaction affects a much greater area, and the local signs are intensified. This response is the immediate reaction, usually occurring within 15–30 min, which serves physiologically to reject the unwelcome antigen and, in superficial sites, to limit its dispersion. In deeper sites, such as muscles, the greater vascularity, aggravated by the increased permeability inherent in the reaction, permits dispersion of the antigen and, presumably, of histamine, 5-hydroxytryptamine and other noxious agents so that a more widespread reaction may occur. In most instances, the reaction is tolerated, with a varying degree of serum sickness according to the amount of local or systemic tissue affected. The immediate local reaction may be masked by dispersion of the antigen or for other immunological reasons, but a delayed reaction begins any time after about 30 min, not infrequently several hours later. Even when the immune response is apparently complete, without clinical sequelae, the process inevitably heightens sensitivity so that a subsequent exposure to penicillin—in any form, at any site—may evoke a more violent reaction. Sensitivity is rapidly increased by repeated stimuli following the cessation of each episode but not if subthreshold doses are injected in rapid succession; this is, in fact, the preferred method of desensitisation. Occasionally, if a long interval elapses without exposure to penicillin, the hypersensitive state may decline or disappear. Alternatively, a stage of extreme hypersensitivity may gradually or suddenly develop, wherein the subject reacts anaphylactically to a small dose, with fall in blood pressure, collapse, coma or convulsions, and death. The reaction of the sensitised subject to a dose of penicillin is therefore extremely variable, depending in the first place upon the route, site, dose and preparation of the drug; and, in the second place, upon the subject himself—his frequency of exposure, degree of sensitivity and constitution, including allergic diathesis. It is virtually impossible to correlate these independent variables into a predictable clinical pattern but it is useful to assess the situation in relation to the drug, the patient and the nature of the reaction.

The drug. The cross-allergenicity of the penicillins has already been mentioned; there is no reliable evidence at present that any penicillin is hypoallergenic in relation to the others. Any dose, however small, may produce a reaction but it is important for everyone including the patient to realise that skin tests with therapeutic penicillins are negative in the majority of sensitised subjects; penicilloyl polylysines (p. 165) are much more likely to give positive results. Topical application causes local pruritis and inflammation echoed in the sites, if any, of primary sensitisation but seldom in sites of subsequent applications of the drug. Intramuscular injection may likewise excite a local reaction; more often this is not obvious and the first signs are general or remote. Intravenous injections may give severe systemic signs but injection by any route, even intradermal, may cause an immediate or delayed systemic reaction, including anaphylaxis. Oral dosage is much less likely to excite or provoke the hypersensitive state but anaphylaxis can, very rarely, occur[45].

The patient may or may not have received penicillin therapeutically; it seems established beyond doubt that some subjects react adversely without having received penicillin as a drug, though they must presumably have been exposed to it in some form: the writer recently witnessed a delayed reaction in a baby, four weeks old, who must have been sensitised *in utero* when his mother, herself hypersensitive, was given penicillin. Frequency of exposure and an allergic diathesis are strong predisposing factors.

References p. 138/139

The reaction may be immediate (0–30 min) or delayed (after 30 min)

Immediate: (*i*) Contact dermatitis

(*ii*) Anaphylaxis (less than 0.1% of all adverse reactions)[46]

Delayed: (*i*) Urticarial skin rashes

(*ii*) Serum sickness

In subjects with an allergic diathesis, the response may be complicated by asthma, eczema, vasomotor rhinitis or other symptoms according to the individual proclivity. In severe delayed reactions, the urticarial changes are not confined to visible parts of the body and there may be a severe though transient general reaction, independent of anaphylaxis. In some instances a particular organ (the "shock organ") may be the target and signs referable to this may dominate all others: in some subjects, not always asthmatic, the lung is the shock organ and dyspnoea the most striking sign; in others, the brain seems to be involved, perhaps by angioedema, and a toxic psychosis with confusion, agitation and disorientation may ensue[47]; in severe cases, or on subsequent occasions, this may worsen to coma, followed by intellectual impairment[48], attributable perhaps to cerebral anoxia during the period of shock.

The reactions may be summarised thus:

Main organ affected	*Reaction*	
	Immediate	*Delayed*
Skin	Pruritus, erythema	Urticaria, dermatitis
Mucosae	Conjunctivitis, stomatitis	Glossitis, laryngeal oedema
Bronchi	Spasm (asthma)	Spasm
Lungs		Oedema, Loeffler's syndrome
Brain		Oedema, anoxia (confusion, convulsion, coma)
Blood vessels	Dilatation, hypotension, shock	Angioedema
Marrow		Neutropenia, eosinophilia, thrombocytopenia
? Kidney		? Haematuria

Any one or several of the above manifestations may appear during an allergic reaction and may be repeated on a subsequent occasion or may occur in changed form. Various complicated syndromes (*e.g.* Stevens–Johnson, polyarteritis) have also been ascribed to penicillin hypersensitivity but these are not proven and it is more likely that they represent exacerbations of preexisting lesions in shock organs. Most experienced investigators find that reactions falsely ascribed to penicillins are much commoner than true reactions, if the following criteria be adopted for confirming a tentative diagnosis:

(*i*) A reaction occurring during penicillin therapy which ceases when the drug is withdrawn.

(*ii*) Is associated with a positive reaction, then or later, to an intradermal injection of penicilloyl polylysine.

(*iii*) Recurs after a subsequent dose of penicillin.

Condition (*iii*) is not justifiable in the case of a patient suffering a severe reaction and is in any case considered only when (*ii*) is negative. Further aspects of the diagnosis and treatment of hypersensitivity are dealt with in Chapter 14.

Idiosyncrasy

A few isolated incidents have recently been reported during therapy with the newer penicillins. These incidents are certainly not due to direct toxicity but have certain features suggestive of hypersensitivity, though none of the patients exhibited any of the other, more characteristic, signs of hypersensitivity described in the section on hypersensitivity above. The most convincing incidents are listed in Table XIV. Hewitt and his colleagues[49], who have wide experience in the use of all the penicillins, noted that three patients receiving moderate doses of methicillin became oliguric between the 14th and 28th days of therapy; the urine contained fresh blood and casts; fever and

TABLE XIV

REPORTS OF TOXICITY* IN THE NEW PENICILLINS

Drug	Toxic signs	Number of cases	Reference
Methicillin	Neutropenia	1	52
Methicillin	Neutropenia	1	53
Methicillin	Oliguria-haematuria	3	49
Methicillin	Oliguria-haematuria	2	51
Methicillin	Oliguria-haematuria	1	50
Methicillin	"Pseudo-infective syndrome"	3	56
Oxacillin	Elevated transaminase	Several	54
Oxacillin	Abnormalities in tests of hepatic function	6	54, 64

* Excluding proved hypersensitivity.

References p. 138/139

eosinophilia were also present. All these signs disappeared when methicillin was discontinued. Only one of these patients was hypersensitive to penicillin but it is known that renal disturbance is extremely rare even in severe allergic reactions. Grattan[50] recorded a similar case, in a child with no known renal abnormality; death occurred subsequently from complications of mucoviscidosis but the kidney at autopsy was normal. In this case, haematuria was provoked at least twice by giving methicillin. In two cases studied by Kirby and his colleagues[51], haematuria was observed during methicillin therapy but the drug was not discontinued and haematuria ceased spontaneously. A sudden fall in the neutrophil granulocytes of the peripheral blood has been observed in a few patients receiving methicillin[52,53] or oxacillin[54]. This occurred in patients not known to be hypersensitive but in each case the dosage was standard and the return to normality very rapid. Granulocytopenia or agranulocytosis is rarely found during allergic reactions but has been recorded[55] and thrombocytopenia is by no means uncommon. In the case reported by McElfresh and Huang[52], the serum-iron concentration rose in a manner suggestive of interference with erythropoiesis. There is no further data concerning these patients and the results of further challenge with penicillins are not recorded. In the only case of this kind seen by the writer, a child with congenital hypoplastic anaemia and haemoglobinopathy, the granulocytes fell and remained below $1000/mm^3$ during methicillin therapy. Dosage, blood levels and excretion were within normal limits. The granulocytes did not return to normal when methicillin was stopped and a subsequent course of methicillin was well-tolerated.

French workers[56] have described "Un syndrome pseudo-infectieux" in patients treated with methicillin. This syndrome consists of a recurrence of pyrexia and malaise in a patient whose infection is, by all other criteria, subsiding. No details are given concerning changes in the blood picture or urine.

The only penicillins connected with these episodes are methicillin and oxacillin. The renal and neutropenic cases have no common features; apart from the possibility of hypersensitivity, there are no clues to the mechanism of these reactions which cannot be due to direct toxicity, since much larger doses of each drug are tolerated for long periods without any evidence of damage or even irritation to the renal tract or bone marrow.

Procaine, esters and additives

These may cause indirect toxicity in various formulations of penicillin G. The only additive commonly used with the newer penicillins is procaine, which effectively allays the pain of injection. This should be added to the methicillin (or other penicillin) at the time of injection, or should be given through the same needle immediately beforehand in doses of 0.5 ml of a 1 % solution. It should not be dispensed with the methicillin for, if the dose is increased, paraesthesia may occur; with large doses, aphasia, transient blindness and psychotic signs may ensue[57].

LOCAL TOXICITY

Any penicillin is locally irritant if excessive amounts are injected into vulnerable sites like the sub-arachnoid space or anterior chamber of the eye. In the sub-arachnoid space or cerebral ventricle, doses of 2–5 mg cause no trouble. In abscess cavities (*e.g.* thoracic empyema), 10–100 mg is non-irritant and gives bactericidal concentrations for 24 h or more. In muscles, 100 mg is often irritant and large doses (500 mg or more) extremely uncomfortable. Continuous administration of large parenteral doses is therefore best given by the intravenous route. Penicillin G is known to interfere with the coagulation of blood if present in high concentration[58]. This could be of importance in local sites, such as dental cavities, but the concentration required (4 mg/ml or more) could be attained during intensive intravenous therapy at the point of cannulation. There is no evidence about the behaviour of the newer penicillins in this respect.

It is clear, from clinical experience and experiment alike, that the penicillin group of drugs is of very limited reactivity toward mammalian cells or, indeed, toward any cells except bacteria. Such reactivity as does exist comes either from the cation, in the case of the salts of penicillanic acid, from the side-chain, or from combination with procaine, esters or oils in long-acting preparations. Protein binding may contribute to indirect toxicity in the form of the irreversible penicillenate or penicilloyl conjugates; the binding to serum proteins is reversible, and of no consequence toxicologically.

The only side-chain showing direct toxicity as yet in man is the isoxazole, which forms metabolites readily; some patients show a rise in serum transaminase which may reflect metabolic activity in the liver. There is no evidence that any damage results from this. Isoxazoles are however more toxic to tissue-cultures than other therapeutic penicillins in use at present. The ethoxynaphthamido side-chain of nafcillin is suspect on theoretical grounds but there is insufficient evidence to disclose whether or not it is toxic in man. All other toxic reactions from penicillins are of the indirect variety. Extension

138 TOXICITY, PHARMACOLOGY

of antimicrobial activity will undoubtedly depend upon introduction of new side-chains but it is to be hoped that this will not introduce toxic groups. For the abolition of allergenicity, modification of the nucleus is more likely to be rewarding, as is shown by the behaviour of cephalosporins.

REFERENCES

1 FLEMING, A., *Brit. J. exp. Path.*, *10* (1929) 226.
2 WELCH, H., PRICE, C. W., NIELSEN, J. K. AND HUNTER, A. C., *J. lab. clin. Med.*, *29* (1944) 809.
3 HAMRE, D. M., RAKE, G., MCKEE, C. M. AND MACPHILLAMY, H. B., *Amer. J. med. Sci.*, *206* (1943) 642.
4 RAKE, G. AND RICHARDSON, A. P., *Ann. N.Y. Acad. Sci.*, *48* (1946) 143.
5 ALSTON, J. M. AND BROOM, J. C., *Brit. med. J.*, *II* (1944) 718.
6 SCHNEIERSON, S. S. AND PERLMAN, E., *Proc. Soc. Exp. Biol.*, *(N.Y.)*, *91* (1956) 229.
7 BOYD, E. M. AND FULFORD, R. A., *Antibiot. Chemother.*, *11*, (1961) 276.
8 DE SOMER, P., VAN DE VOORDE, H., EYSSEN, H. AND VAN-DIJCKI, P., *Antibiot. Chemother. 5* (1955) 463.
9 CARLSON, S. AND WALKER, C., *Arch. Hyg. (Berl.)*, *147* (1963) 201.
10 LOEWE, L., ROSENBLATT, P. AND ALTURE-WERBER, E., *Amer. Heart. J.*, *32* (1946) 327.
11 BIGBY, MARY A. M. AND JONES, F. AVERY, *J. Obstr. Gynaec. Brit. Emp.*, *56* (1949) 636–647.
12 SPITZY, K. H., *Arzneimittelforsch.*, *12* (1962) 172.
13 BRANCH, A., RODGER, K. C., LEE, R. W. AND POWER, E. E., *Canad. med. Assoc. J.*, *83* (1960) 991.
14 HEWITT, W. L., *J. Amer. med. Assoc.*, *185* (1963) 264.
15 CALLAGHAN, R. P., COHEN, S. J. AND STEWART, G. T., *Brit. med. J.*, *I* (1961) 860.
16 STEWART, G. T., *Pharmakotherapia, 1* (1963) 197.
17 IVLER, D., THRUPP, L. D., LEEDOM, J. M., WEHRLE, P. F. AND PORTNOY, B., *Antimicrobial Agents and Chemotherapy*, (1963) 335.
18 KENNEDY, R. P., PERKINS, J. C. AND JACKSON, G. G., *Antimicrobial Agents and Chemotherapy*, (1962) 506.
19 ABRAHAM, E. P., FLETCHER, C. M., FLOREY, H. W., GARDNER, A. D., HEATLEY, N. G. AND JENNINGS, M. A., *Lancet, ii* (1941) 177.
20 RAUTZ, L. A. AND KIRBY, W. M. M., *J. clin. Invest.*, *23* (1944) 789.
21 EAGLE, H. AND MUSSALMAN, A. D., *Science*, *103* (1946) 618.
22 EAGLE, H. AND NEWMAN, E. V., *J. clin. Invest.*, *26* (1947) 903.
23 COLVILLE, J. M. AND QUINN, E. L., *Antimicrobial Agents and Chemotherapy*, (1961) 600.
24 BEYER, K. H., MILLER, A. K., RUSSO, H. F., PATCH, E. A. AND VERWEY, W. F., *Amer. J. Physiol.*, *149* (1947) 355.
25 STEVENSON, G. H. AND HARRISON, K. JOY, *Brit. med. J.*, *II* (1960) 1596.
26 ACRED, P. AND BROWN, D. M., *Brit. J. Pharmacol.*, *21* (1963) 339.
27 STEWART, G. T. AND HARRISON, PATRICIA M., *Brit. J. Pharmacol.*, *17* (1961) 414.
28 ACRED, P., BROWN, D. M., TURNER, D. H. AND WRIGHT, D., *Brit. J. Pharmacol.*, *18* (1962) 356.
29 RANDALL, W. A., WELCH, H. AND PRICE, C. W., *J. Amer. Pharm. Assoc.*, *36* (1947) 17.
30 GARROD, L. P. AND WATERWORTH, PAMELA M., *Brit. Heart J.*, *24* (1962) 39.

31 STEWART, G. T., COLES, H. M. T., NIXON, H. H. AND HOLT, R. J., *Brit. med. J.*, *II* (1961) 200.
32 ENGLISH, A. R., HUANG, H. T. AND SOBIN, B. A., *Proc. Soc. exp. Biol. (N.Y.)*, *104* (1960) 405.
33 ISENBERG, H. D., PISANO, M. A., CARITO, S. L. AND BERKMAN, J. I., *Antibiot. Chemother.*, *10* (1960) 353.
34 SIEBURGH, J., MCNEILL, A. AND ROTH, F. J., *J. Bact.*, *67* (1954) 460.
35 GALE, D. AND SANDOVAL, B., *J. Bact.*, *75* (1957) 616.
36 GRASSET, E. AND FLEURY, C., *Praxis*, *42* (1953) 285.
37 SHARP, J. L., *Lancet*, *i* (1954) 390.
38 STEWART, G. T., *Brit. med. J.*, *I* (1956) 658.
39 LUPIN, A. M., DASCOMB, H. E., SEABURY, J. H. AND MCGINN, M., *Antimicrobial Agents and Chemotherapy* (1961) 10.
40 VINNICOMBE, J., *Lancet*, *i* (1962) 1186.
41 RITTENBURY, M. S., HUME, D. M. AND HENCH, M., *Antimicrobial Agents and Chemotherapy*, (1962) 51.
42 GUTHE, T., IDSOE, O. AND WILLCOX, R. R., *Bull. Wld. Hlth. Org.*, *19* (1958) 427.
43 HOIGNE, R., *Acta Allerg. (Kbh.)*, *17* (1962) 521.
44 TRINCA, J. C., *Med. J. Australia*, *2* (1962) 428.
45 LEVINE, M. I., PERRI, J. AND ANTHONY, J. J., *J. Allergy*, *31* (1960) 487.
46 ANDERSEN, N. A., *Med. J. Australia*, *1* (1959) 877.
47 COHEN, S. B., *J. Psychiat.*, *11* (1955) 699.
48 COHEN, S. B., *J. Amer. med. Assoc.*, *186* (1963) 899.
49 HEWITT, W. L., FINEGOLD, S. M. AND MOUZOU, O. T., *Antimicrobial Agents and Chemotherapy*, (1961) 765.
50 GRATTAN, W. A., *J. Pediat.*, *64* (1964) 285.
51 ALLEN, J. D., ROBERTS, C., EVANS, J. AND KIRBY, W. M. M., *New Eng. J. Med.*, *266* (1962) 111.
52 MCELFRESH, A. E. AND HUANG, NANCY, *New Eng. J. Med.*, *266* (1962) 246.
53 BULLOCK, W. E., *Antimicrobial Agents and Chemotherapy*, (1961) 770.
54 *Medical Letter*, *4* (1962) 29.
55 SIGAL, E. S., *Kazan med. Zh.*, *1* (1963) 59.
56 VIC-DUPONT, RAPIN, M. AND HUALT, G., *Presse méd.*, *71* (1963) 271.
57 BJORNBERG, A. AND SELSTAM, J., *Acta Psych. Scand.*, *35* (1960) 129.
58 FLEMING, A. AND FISH, E. W., *Brit. med. J.*, *II* (1947) 242.
59 GREENBERG, H. L. AND RUTENBERG, A. M., *Antimicrobial Agents and Chemotherapy*, (1962) 779.
60 HOLLOWAY, W. J., PETERS, C. D., AND SCOTT, E. G., *Antimicrobial Agents and Chemotherapy*, (1961) 314.
61 BEARGIE, R. A., AND RILEY, H. D., *Antimicrobial Agents and Chemotherapy*, (1963) 331.
62 CHRISTIE, A. B., *Brit. med. J.*, *I* (1964) 1609.
63 ROSENTHAL, J. M., ADAMS, B. W. AND METZGER, W. I., *Antimicrobial Agents and Chemotherapy*, (1963) 227.
64 TEN PAS, A. AND QUINN, E. L., *J. Amer. med. Assoc.*, *191* (1965) 674.

Chapter 13

RESISTANCE TO THE PENICILLINS

There is reason to believe (see Chapter 9) that penicillin G and possibly some other derivatives of 6-APA act upon all bacteria, though only certain species or strains are sufficiently affected to be susceptible *in vivo* to therapeutic concentrations. The term "resistance" is therefore to some extent arbitrary, connoting either insusceptibility of the organism to a therapeutic level of the drug or a sensitivity markedly less than that of the average bacterial cell of the same species. For laboratory purposes it is not difficult to define an arbitrary standard concentration and to express drug-resistance as increments above this; for clinical purposes the same definitions do not necessarily apply, especially since most of the penicillins are non-toxic within wide limits. The purpose of the present chapter is to examine the problem of resistance from the clinical and epidemiological viewpoints; resistance induced by laboratory procedures will be considered only in so far as it affects this larger problem.

Penicillin-resistant bacteria may be divided into two broad categories:

NATURAL OR INHERENT RESISTANCE

Organisms in this category contain populations of cells which are uniformly unaffected by high concentrations of the drugs in question. That is to say, these organisms are morphologically unchanged and can multiply at an approximately normal rate in nutrient media containing concentrations upwards of 20 μg/ml, the exact level being dependent upon the level of drug ordinarily attained and maintained in the usual sites of infection appropriate to the particular organism. The mechanisms of resistance and the degree of resistance exhibited by organisms within this category vary, and there is a broad overlap with certain other categories which may be deemed, for the moment, relatively sensitive. Various factors are involved in the insusceptibility: drug-stable metabolism, impenetrability of the cell, destruction of the drug, and other factors.

ACQUIRED RESISTANCE

This implies the acquisition by individual bacterial cells or whole populations of powers of growth in concentrations hitherto inhibitory or bactericidal. In the laboratory, such resistance is readily produced in many bacterial species by exposure to the drug. In human beings such strains seem to arise either by replacing drug-sensitive bacterial populations during therapy or prophylaxis, or by inducing resistance in successive generations of cells originating from a sensitive parent.

There are at present three main theories about the origin and mechanism of resistance, as follows:

(1) *Mutation.* Spontaneous genotypical changes are known to occur during multiplication of organisms, and are generally held to explain variation of a species. The acquisition of drug-resistance is a particular example of this natural and inevitable phenomenon[1,2] which may occur without exposure to the drug though the presence of the drug favours propagation of the mutant by eliminating competitors. Mutants may transfer their resistance to sensitive cells by sexual recombination of nuclear material, as in *Esch. coli* K. 12 (ref. 3), in which resistance is controlled by one or more genes[4]. Such transfer may be effected by DNA extracts[5], in which case it is known as *transformation*, or by *transduction* by phages acting upon the organisms[6]. The natural rate of mutation in bacteria is known to be low[7] (10^{-5}–10^{-10}) and, even if irradiation and other artificial agents increase this rate, antibacterial drugs do not appear to do so directly. Not all organisms showing mutational resistance have been studied in detail, but there is some evidence[8] that, in *E. coli* at least, the genes controlling resistance are arranged in a linear sequence of known order; in brief, mutation means the loss or change of one of these genes.

(2) *Adaptation.* In contrast, this is a non-genetic change due to cytoplasmic alterations in the bacterial cell. This theory requires a Lamarckian assumption that the metabolism of cells can be progressively if not permanently altered by physico-chemical adaptation. On biochemical grounds, the theory might well be valid[9]; with regard to drug-resistance, the only proved example of adaptation is the acquisition of resistance to penicillin by *B. cereus*[10] and *Staph. aureus*[11] by induction of penicillinase. In the case of *Staph. aureus* it is very probable that induction is non-genic, residing in a cytoplasmic determinant[12]. Drug-resistance due to organisms of lesser sensitivity persisting after the elimination of the majority of cells in a predominantly-sensitive bacterial population may be another instance of adaptation. The importance of

these "persisters" has been thoroughly examined by McDermott[13] who pointed out that recognition of the phenomenon "was not possible before the introduction of penicillin" and that the identification of latent or persisting organisms in the tissues is one of the few indisputably-proved manifestations of clinical resistance to chemotherapy.

(3) *Episomal resistance.* Fragments of nuclear material, known as episomes, may exist free in the chromosomes or cytoplasm[14]. If these originate from that part of the chromosome containing the genic factors responsible for drug-resistance, they may pass from generation to generation, converting sensitive organisms by cell-to-cell contact without nuclear recombination.

As the result of the operation of these mechanisms, resistance to drugs may develop in various stages and patterns. The simplest form is the obligatory one-step pattern in which the bacterial population contains only one type of highly resistant mutant. If these mutants are present together with others which develop resistance more gradually, and variable in degree, the pattern is known as one-step/multi-step, typical of that found with streptomycin and isoniazid[7]. When the mutants are all of low-resistance, repeated exposure to the drug is required to select out the populations with potentially higher resistance, which therefore develops in a multi-step pattern. This is typical of resistance to penicillin. With certain organisms, adaptive and episomal mechanisms may interplay with mutation to produce more complicated patterns of resistance.

BIOCHEMICAL FACTORS IN PENICILLIN RESISTANCE

It is a fascinating if thankless thought that penicillins are the only therapeutic substances which act as specific substrates for inactiving enzymes (penicillinases) of bacterial origin. One of these enzymes, β-lactamase, seems to be designed with uncanny precision to fit the penicillin (and cephalosporin) molecule; the other enzyme, amidase, probably attacks penicillins as well as other substrates.

β-Lactamase

The enzyme formed by staphylococci naturally resistant to penicillin G is invariably a β-lactamase (Fig. 9), opening the lactam ring hydrolytically to convert the active benzyl penicillins to the corresponding inactive penicil-

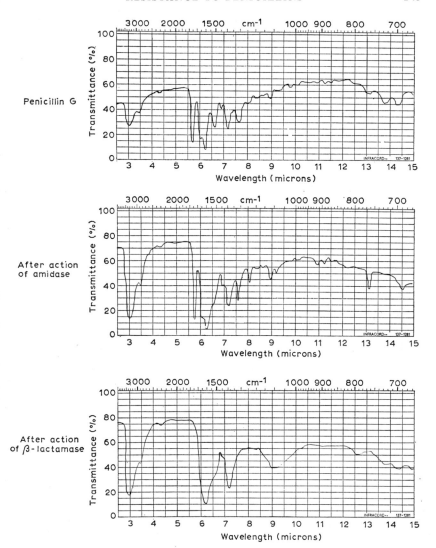

Fig. 9. Effect of amidase and β-lactamase on penicillin G. The absorption peak in the 5.5–6.0 μ band (1760 cm^{-1}), characteristic of the carbonyl group in the intact lactam ring, is retained after exposure of penicillin G to amidase but lost after exposure to β-lactamase. The readings were made on a recording infrared spectrophotometer before and after exposure of the drug to bacterial cells producing the respective enzymes.

loic acids[15]. β-lactamase with an identical action in terms of end-products, in also formed by various coliforms, *Bact. aerogenes*, *B. subtilis* and *B. cereus*[16], among other organisms, though the production of the enzyme is a feature of species or strains and not of whole genera with the possible exception of *B. cereus*[17] in which a genetic factor connected with the production of the enzyme may always be present. β-lactamase may be formed *constitutively*, by bacteria growing in the absence of substrate, or *inducibly*, *i.e.* only in response to the presence of substrate. As Pollock[18] has pointed out, three stages are then necessary for the occurrence of resistance due to enzyme-formation: first, the bacterial cell must acquire the necessary genetic information for production of the enzyme; secondly, substrate must be present for specific induction; and thirdly, environmental conditions must be appropriate for hydrolysis. In coliforms, *Bact. aerogenes* and other gram-negative bacilli, powerful inactivating enzymes are formed constitutively[19], in *Staph. aureus*, the basal level of enzyme-production may be insufficient to protect the organism from the drug but under conditions of induction[18] full resistance is exhibited. Wild strains of *B. cereus* produce the enzyme inducibly but mutants derived from these strains produce it constitutively[20]. Two such mutants of *B. cereus* (569 and 5B) produce potent exo-cellular β-lactamases[21,22] which have been characterised and used extensively to investigate hydrolysis of the various penicillins; such results are of undoubted interest theoretically but, from the clinical viewpoint, it has to be remembered that both enzyme and substrate are used in most of these studies in artificially-high concentrations and that *B. cereus* is not a pathogen. *Staph. aureus* also forms an exo-enzyme which has now been purified[23]; it has a molecular weight of 29,600 and contains 41 % by weight of aspartic acid and lysine which is present as the N-terminal amino acid probably in a single polypeptide chain; this enzyme also exhibits specific activity against the cephalosporin molecule, probably accounting for all the so-called "cephalosporinase" activity reported in staphylococcal culture filtrates[24].

The site of action of staphylococcal β-lactamase upon the penicillin molecule is affected by the steric configuration of certain hindered side-chains such as the dimethoxybenzamido (in methicillin) and the various 3-phenyl-4-isoxazolyl substituents. These side-chains are less effective however in interfering with the action of β-lactamase produced by other organisms such as *B. cereus*, coliforms and *Bact. aerogenes*[25-27]. Hence, while methicillin and its analogues can resist inactivation by staphylococci, they are less well equipped to withstand these other species[28] which may be present in mixed infections or commensally in the intestine.

The outcome of the reaction between any penicillin (or cephalosporin) and β-lactamase *in vivo* is extremely difficult to assess. *In vitro*, conditions can be standardised and experiments have shown that the affinity of the substrate for the enzyme, inducibility of the latter, rate of hydrolysis and, not least, the initial bactericidal effect of the drug, all contribute individually to the result. Methicillin probably owes its efficacy, *in vivo* as well as in the test tube, to low affinity (*Km* with staphylococcal β-lactamase 12,000 times higher than with penicillin G) and low rate of hydrolysis (V_{max} 30 times less than with penicillin G)[18]. This means that, at equivalent concentrations, methicillin has a half-life 360,000 times longer than that of penicillin G in the presence of an active β-lactamase-forming staphylococcus[27]. So far, the enzymes from staphylococci have been uniformly inert towards methicillin but, by analogy with the *Bacillus* species, it is conceivable that a further mutation or genic recombination might promote the production of a different β-lactamase; it is very important that strains of staphylococci resistant to methicillin and its analogues be investigated carefully in relation to this possibility (see p. 180), even though, on the basis of present information, the resistance of these strains is not attributable to any kind of inactivating enzyme (Fig. 10).

Amidase

The other site in the penicillin molecule amenable to enzymatic hydrolysis is the peptide linkage in the 6-position:

$$R{-}CO{-}NH\text{---}\overset{S}{\diagdown}(Me)_2 + H_2O \rightleftharpoons R{\cdot}COOH + NH_2\text{---}\overset{S}{\diagdown}(Me)_2$$

carboxylic acid   6-APA

If this is split, the penicillin is deacylated and 6-APA formed as an end-product. Unlike penicilloic acids, 6-APA has weak antibacterial activity, especially against gram-negative bacilli; so inactivation is less complete than with β-lactamase. Various micro-organisms form amidases capable of partially inactivating penicillins by deacylation, including moulds such as *Penicillium* itself, various yeasts and actinomycetes, notably *Str. lavendulae*[29] which hydrolyses penicillin V more readily than penicillin G. These enzymes give up to 56% of the theoretical yield of 6-APA, act optimally at 50° at pH 9.0; the end-product 6-APA limits the reaction at a concentration of 4.0 mg/ml. The reverse reaction, with resynthesis of a benzyl penicillin, proceeds if the pH is lowered to 5.0–5.5. Various bacteria, including coliforms and many

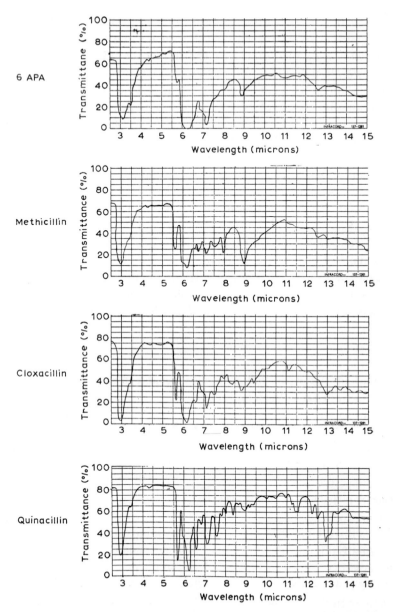

Fig. 10. Effect of β-lactamase on various penicillins. The lactam ring of 6-APA (absorption peak in the 5.5–6.0 μ band) is extinguished by exposure to the enzyme. Methicillin, cloxacillin and quinacillin are unaffected. (See Fig. 9).

gram-negative bacilli, but not the pyogenic cocci or other gram-positive species, also form amidase[28,30]. *E. coli* forms amidase more often than β-lactamase and the enzyme from this, which is partly exo-cellular, has been partially purified[31]. Unlike the enzyme produced by fungi, this amidase acts hydrolytically at pH 5–8 at 40°. It also attacks penicillin V, ampicillin and cephalosporins. Hydrolysis of penicillins G or V by amidase is now used for the commercial production of 6-APA.

Whereas β-lactamase is often, sometimes only, formed inducibly, amidase appears to be essentially a constitutive enzyme. It has been suggested[28] that all bacteria form some kind of amidase, probably as part of a non-specific peptidase essential for metabolism and growth. Peptide substrates such as leucinamide are therefore hydrolysed readily but amidases with specific activity against penicillins (penamidase) seem to be confined to certain gram-negative bacilli and this is undoubtedly one factor in the lesser susceptibility which these organisms generally show toward the penicillins. The side-chain can interfere with the action of amidase, which is sterically close to that of β-lactamase. If methicillin is exposed to amidase followed by β-lactamase it is more readily inactivated than by either enzyme alone[28]. Amidase-production does not confer the high degree of resistance to penicillin G which is possessed by organisms forming β-lactamase; it is a less powerful enzyme, inactivation is incomplete and the end-product (6-APA) not only limits the reaction but itself retains some antibacterial potency.

In practical terms, amidase is important only in relation to commensal and pathogenic gram-negative bacilli. Commensal organisms capable of forming amidase are present in the intestine, and may colonise the absorptive part of the small intestine and the oropharynx during oral therapy with penicillins. This might result in diminution of therapeutic potency prior to absorption; free 6-APA, presumably resulting from this process, has been detected in the urine of a patient receiving penicillin V[32] though, in the writer's experience, this must be extremely rare. Pathogenic organisms like *E. coli, Proteus* spp. and others may or may not form amidase but, if they do, they are likely to be more resistant for that reason to ampicillin; they may also resist the action of some cephalosporin derivatives.

These inactivating enzymes are undoubtedly factors in the resistance of various bacteria to the penicillins but they are not the only ones and not always dominant. In the case of *Staph. aureus*, the rapid production of a powerful β-lactamase probably explains the complete resistance which can defy therapy with the older penicillins but the organism has to grow to form enzyme and a small inoculum can be killed or inhibited before this occurs.

References p. 157/158

When enzyme is being formed, the presence of penicillin acts as an inducer. Gram-negative bacilli, having lower inherent susceptibility, are better able to survive to form either enzyme. There are important differences between the penicillinases of gram-positive and gram-negative origin, the latter being more diverse, constitutive and differently treated in the cell; their activation energy is also lower[33]. Amidase produced only by gram-negative bacilli is less important but the genetic and adaptive mechanisms responsible for the conversion of the ubiquitous, non-specific forms of this enzyme into specific penamidase are undefined and in need of further study.

RESISTANCE OF INDIVIDUAL BACTERIA

Staphylococci

Not all of the mechanisms outlined above apply to the penicillins. Laboratory multi-step mutants of staphylococci have high intrinsic resistance but form no penicillinase[34] whereas resistant strains isolated from hospital patients often have low intrinsic resistance but always produce penicillinase (refs. 35–37) and usually belong to phage group III or to certain types within group I[38]. If a strain of *Staph. aureus* (coagulase-positive) is sensitive to a penicillin when isolated from a patient, treatment of that patient with that penicillin does not result in acquisition of drug-resistance by the organism. This does not apply to *Staph. albus* (coagulase-negative) which may develop resistance to penicillin G, methicillin or the isoxazole penicillins during treatment[39]. With both types of staphylococci, clinical resistance to penicillin G is undoubtedly due to a progressive increase in the prevalence of penicillinase-forming strains which existed in small numbers before the advent of penicillin[40], and became predominant quickly in hospital communities more or less in proportion to the therapeutic usage of penicillin. Such strains spread mainly by cross-infection. Their incidence within hospitals is therefore high; outside hospitals, it is low but not negligible, for strains acquired by out-patients can spread within families and closed communities. The original source of these penicillinase-forming strains is speculative: it might seem remarkable that certain micro-organisms should be provided in advance with an enzyme designed specifically to hydrolyse a unique lactam-ring structure unknown elsewhere in nature; but it should be remembered that penicillin-forming moulds are common on cheese and other decaying foodstuffs where organisms such as staphylococci, *B. cereus*, *B. subtilis* and coliforms (all penicillinase-formers) are also abundant. Recent work from New Zealand[41] offers an intriguing ecological clue to this riddle of nature: hedgehogs there are habitually infected with dermatophytes (*Trichophyton mentagrophytes* or similar species) which produce sufficient penicillinase to preclude secondary staphylococcal infection except by penicillinase-forming strains!

Resistance of staphylococci to the newer penicillins
   Methicillin, the isoxazole penicillins and other derivatives with hindered side-chains are insusceptible to staphylococcal penicillinase (β-lactamase) and the great majority of strains of *Staph. aureus*, irrespectively of origin, are therefore sensitive to these drugs. Resistant strains do however occur, though rarely as yet. The power to control staphylococcal infection depends largely upon the continuing efficacy of these drugs, so it is important to examine the

TABLE XV

PRIMARY ISOLATIONS OF STAPHYLOCOCCI RESISTANT TO THE NEWER PENICILLINS

Ref.	Number of strains	Place	Source	Active or passive infection	Phage group		Number of patients affected
42	1	England	Carrier	Passive	III (7, 47, 53, 54, 75, 77)		1
61	1	England	Bedsore	Doubtful	III (53, 54, 75, 77)		1
43	1	England	Lesions and carrier sites	Both	III (75, 77+)	1 fatality (post-operative)	37
44	1	England	Lesions	Active	III		5
45	2	England	Lesions	Active	III	Fatal case	1
49	3	Denmark	Lesions and carrier sites	Both	III		3
48	1	Poland	Carrier-sites	Passive	III (untypeable)		20
46	9	England Switzerland South Africa Egypt	Lesions and carrier sites Also objects	Both	Mainly III various types	27,479 strains tested for methicillin-resistance	Uncertain
51	7	Canada	3 lesions 4 carrier-sites	Both	I 80/82, 81/82 81 II 3A, 3B, 55/71 III 83A/53 42E/73		

TABLE XVI

NUMBER OF CHILDREN EACH MONTH HARBOURING METHICILLIN-RESISTANT *Staph. aureus*

Ward	Mar	Apr.	May	June	July	Aug.	Sept.	Oct.	Nov.	Dec.	Jan.	Feb.	Mar.	Apr.	May
Number of children with resistant strain of Staphylococcus (1961–62)															
E1 Acute med. (babies)	2	3	1	5	3	1	2	1	1	1		1	3	2	1
E2 Acute med. (babies)				1											
B2 Acute med.					1	1	1						1	1	1
B4 Acute surg. (babies)									2				1	1	1
D2 Orthopaedic									1						
B7 Gastroenteritis												1	1	1	
B3 Acute med.													1	1	4
F4 Acute med.															1
Other wards (40)															
Ward staff												1			
Total cases	2	3	1	6	4	2	3	1	4	1	—	3	7	6	8*
No. of patients in hospital (weekly averages)	472		481			465			606		657	683	675	667	65

* Fatal case.

Reproduced from the *British Medical Journal*, *I* (1963) 308, by kind permission of the Editor.

origin and nature of these new resistant strains. After the introduction of methicillin for clinical use, some months passed before the first resistant strain was isolated[42]. This strain—the only one showing resistance out of about 10,000 tested within that period—was unconnected with therapy; the resistant cells were a minority of the total, were slow-growing, atypical and probably avirulent. In succeeding months, similar strains appeared here and there but there was no evidence of increase, of any connection with therapy, or of invasiveness (Table XV). Then, in a hospital where methicillin was first used in 1959, a resistant strain was isolated from a nasal carrier in 1961 and gradually spread (Table XVI) to other patients and other wards throughout the hospital[43]. Between 1959 and 1961, methicillin had been used intensively and all staphylococci isolated or re-isolated from patients had been tested; other penicillins (propicillin, isoxazole derivatives, ampicillin) were also being tested but resistance was never observed as a result of therapy and the resistant strains, when eventually isolated, were not connected with therapy with any of these newer penicillins, though many of the patients had received penicillin G or V. In the succeeding year, the resistant strain (type 75, 77, +)

was isolated on 71 occasions from 37 patients, not more than 2% of the population at risk being affected at the point of maximal incidence. Most of the patients carried the organism passively; a few minor lesions occurred and there was one fatality: a child who was receiving methicillin and strepto-mycin prophylactically developed a wound infection followed by septicae-mia; this child was in a vulnerable state after a neurosurgical operation but the fact that the resistant organism was acquired during methicillin prophy-laxis and that it was isolated from disseminated lesions post-mortem showed that it was virulent. Thereafter the resistant strain disappeared spontaneous-ly. Isolated incidents demonstrating the virulence of resistant strains have been recorded in other centres[44,45]. Of 27,479 strains of *Staph. aureus* sent to the reference laboratory at Colindale, 102 were methicillin-resistant[46]; these strains came from hospitals in places as far apart as England, Switzer-land, Egypt and South Africa and were temporarily endemic in at least two hospitals. A later minor epidemic in Poland[47] showed again that resistant strains could appear without methicillin being used therapeutically and could occur in different types of staphylococci.

The strains of *Staph. aureus* which are resistant to methicillin show some important common properties: they are all relatively resistant to all other penicillins and probably to some derivatives of cephalosporin; they are all strong penicillinase-formers but they do not owe their resistance to this fact, for they do not inactivate methicillin appreciably and their enzyme (β-lac-tamase) is serologically identical with that formed by methicillin-sensitive staphylococci of the same phage patterns[48]. According to some workers, the β-lactamase from these strains may be sufficiently powerful to inactivate the isoxazole penicillins at therapeutic concentrations[43], or even to inactivate methicillin[49] but, whether or not this is the case, it is clear that the resistance of the organisms is not due to the enzyme. Most resistant strains are resistant also to other antibiotics, especially tetracycline, and to mercury; some of the Polish strains are resistant also to phenyl–methane dyes like gentian violet, though this property, like mercury resistance, occurs also in methicillin-sensitive staphylococci. The individual bacterial cells are swollen in the pres-ence of methicillin but this is corrected by the addition of 6% sodium chlo-ride to the medium[50], indicating that methicillin may be permitting osmotic distension of the cell substance by affecting the cell wall or inner cytoplasmic membrane.

Epidemiologically, there is an unexplained anomaly in the fact that very few strains have been found in North America, even in centres where an intensive search has been conducted[51]. The absence of resistant strains in

References p. 157/158

North America, where all the newer penicillins are widely used, contrasted with their presence in Poland, where the new derivatives of 6-APA are not available, provides definite proof that the occurrence of resistant staphylococci does not depend upon the therapeutic use of methicillin and its analogues. Epidemiologically and otherwise, the problem of staphylococcal resistance to the newer penicillins is therefore different from the penicillinase-type resistance which compromised the therapeutic status of penicillin G. For practical purposes, this difference is important. Patients harbouring these strains should of course be isolated, treated and discharged from hospital as quickly as possible. There is no indication at present that methicillin or the isoxazole derivatives should be restricted in use for this reason; indeed, where methicillin has been used most widely and intensively, as in the routine spraying of wards affected by heavy staphylococcal cross-infection, no resistance whatsoever has been encountered[25,52,53]. This may be because few of the strains are highly resistant and since some contain only a minority of resistant cells in their population. In this event methicillin in large doses might even serve to eliminate the resistant organisms and establish by its very use a self-regulatory mechanism akin to the suppression by penicillin G of *Str. pyogenes*.

Streptococci

There is no authentic record of natural resistance to penicillin G on the part of streptococci of group A, either on primary isolation or after therapy, even if prolonged. The continuing efficacy of penicillin prophylaxis in rheumatic fever after many years is in itself proof of this. With the exception of ampicillin, the newer penicillins are less active against these organisms than penicillins G or V, and are therefore not used except for specific therapy unless another organism is present. Resistance can be induced *in vitro* but there is no record of it occurring *in vivo*, or of strains showing any significant degree of resistance at first isolation.

Streptococci of other groups, including anaerobic streptococci, vary in sensitivity to all penicillins except ampicillin, which inhibits most species at 5 μg/ml or less, usually much less. *Str. viridans*, enterococci and non-haemolytic streptococci are often inherently resistant to methicillin and the isoxazole derivatives, and sometimes to penicillin G. During therapy and especially during prolonged prophylaxis with any penicillin, sensitive streptococci disappear from the pharynx and resistant streptococci appear but whether this is replacement or acquisition of resistance is never clear, for organisms of these species cannot be accurately typed. Induced resistance is however uncommon in the prolonged treatment of endocarditis due to *Str. viridans* or *Str. faecalis*.

Pneumococcus

This organism behaves like the group A streptococcus. All authentic strains are sensitive to penicillin G and, in lesser degree, to the newer penicillins, and resistance has not been observed during treatment. A few unusual strains have recently been isolated in Edinburgh (Calder, personal communication) which are resistant to 1 μg/ml of penicillin G. These strains have the capsular antigens of pneumococci but are atypical in that they are not inhibited by optochin or soluble in bile.

Gonococcus

Though normally extremely sensitive, the gonococcus can develop resistance to penicillin G (up to 1 μg/ml) and it is now established that resistance even of this relatively low order militates against successful therapy[54]. The only newer derivative employed in the treatment of gonorrhoea is ampicillin, which appears to be moderately successful[55,56], but it is too early to judge whether or not resistance will be a problem with this drug. Its action however is so similar to that of penicillin G that resistance seems a likelihood.

Meningococcus

This organism is highly sensitive to ampicillin, which can be used instead of penicillin G or sulphonamides in the treatment of meningitis (see p. 61). It is insufficiently sensitive to the other new penicillins to warrant their use in therapy. There are no reports of drug-resistance.

Proteus species

These organisms are inherently resistant to all penicillins except ampicillin and, to a lesser degree, penicillin G, to which many strains of *P. mirabilis* and some strains of *P. vulgaris* are sensitive. If the organism is not eliminated quickly in therapy, drug-resistance of a fairly high order can develop (see p. 55). Some strains form amidase, others form β-lactamase, but resistance, inherent or acquired, may be present independently of these enzymes. Strains

References p. 157/158

spreading in hospital by cross-infection (*e.g.* in patients with chronic urinary disorders) are, more often than not, too resistant to ampicillin for therapy with this drug to be contemplated.

Coliforms

Like *Proteus*, this group of organisms is highly resistant to methicillin, the isoxazoles, nafcillin, quinacillin and, for practical purposes, penicillin G. Some strains of *E. coli*, paracolon bacilli and related species are inhibited by ampicillin in attainable concentrations (2–20 μg/ml) but resistance, or super-infection by closely-related resistant strains, may occur during therapy though less readily than with *Proteus*. Many strains form amidase or β-lactamase, and high resistance is often due to the production of these enzymes (p. 142).

Klebsiella-aerogenes

This large and diverse group of bacteria is, in general, inherently resistant to all forms of penicillin, though occasionally strains are isolated which are moderately sensitive to ampicillin (10–20 μg/ml). Faecal strains of *Bact. aerogenes* are among the most resistant of all bacteria, often due to the production of a powerful, constitutive β-lactamase.

Pseudomonas pyocyanea

This organism, like other species of *Pseudomonas*, is inherently resistant to all forms of penicillin whether or not inactivating enzymes are formed. As a matter of academic interest, strains are sometimes encountered which are feebly inhibited by derivatives of 6-APA with a free amino group like ampicillin or *p*-aminobenzyl penicillin (50 μg/ml). No derivative of 6-APA so far described has any stronger action, so the *Pseudomonas* group of organisms remains as a major gap in the spectrum of penicillins.

Salmonella

Like most other gram-negative bacilli, this large group is primarily resistant to methicillin and all the penicillinase-stable penicillins; there is, in fact, a paradoxical correlation between penicillinase stability and inactivity against gram-negative bacilli (see Chapter 10). With the exception of *S. typhimurium*, most members of the *Salmonella* group are sensitive to penicillin G and, more consistently, to ampicillin which may find an increasing place in the treatment of carriers of these organisms[57]. Increased resistance has not so far been reported during or after the treatment of cases or carriers, despite intensive testing of re-isolated strains. *Salmonellae* do not form amidase or β-lactamase.

Shigellae

The various members of this group are usually resistant to the penicillins but a proportion of strains of *Sh. flexneri* and *Sh. sonnei* are inhibited by ampicillin (5 μg/ml) and may be eradicated from chronic carriers by treatment with this drug[58]. Resistance has not been noted in re-isolated strains.

Haemophilus

This organism is regularly sensitive only to ampicillin, which has been used in long-term chemoprophylaxis or therapy of chronic bronchitis. Drug-resistance has not been reported.

Other organisms

Many other pathogens show varying degrees of inherent resistance to some of the newer penicillins, especially to methicillin and quinacillin, which have extremely narrow antibacterial spectra. Apart from the organisms specified above, there are very few indications for the preferential use of the newer derivatives and there is therefore no data concerning the development of drug-resistance by other organisms, though it is known that most genera can acquire resistance by selection of mutants or adaptation during passage in laboratory media.

In academic circles, resistance to penicillin has provoked about as much interest as therapy. It is to be hoped that what is lacking in knowledge about countering resistance is balanced by the mass of genetic and enzymological data which has thereby accumulated. Apart from steric hindrance, which partly accounts for the stability of methicillin and its analogues to penicillinase, there are no certain leads to the prevention of resistance. From the preceding paragraphs, it is clear that there are many other factors besides penicillinase in resistance, especially in so far as it impedes or threatens the therapeutic usefulness of the newer derivatives.

This is not to say that the problem is insoluble. Certain broad leads have not as yet been intensively explored. The penicillins are without exception much more active against gram-positive cocci than against gram-negative bacilli; this orientation of activity is strongly correlated with: (*a*) Insusceptibility to penicillinase: the more selective the action on gram-positive species, the greater the stability to both amidase and β-lactamase. This indicates a connection in terms of chemical charge or structure, between the sites of gram-positive activity and enzyme-attachment. (*b*) Gram-positive potency is largely dependent upon interruption of mucopeptide synthesis by a biochemical pathway which is less vital in the cell walls of gram-negative bacilli; gram-negativity is by itself an irrelevant property, for some gram-negative cocci are the most sensitive of all species. (*c*) Gram-negative activity is heightened by free basic groups at various sites in the acyl side-chain.

Irrespectively of the gram-difference, or even of species, susceptibility of an organism to low concentrations of penicillin is associated with interference with cell-wall synthesis, and probably some binding at specific receptor sites. It has been suggested that organisms, even relatively resistant organisms, may have a single "portal of entry"[59] which governs the effective access of penicillin G at least to the penicillinase-inducing centre and to the locus of action on the cell wall which may in turn be related to the "penicillin-binding centre" of Cooper and Rowley[60]. Information on these matters is largely based on experiments with penicillin G; there is a need for a repeat and extension of this work with the newer derivatives and with 6-APA itself, differentially labelled by isotopes to indicate the role of the side-chain.

From the practical viewpoint, genetic studies have so far been unhelpful. They have yielded much information which would favour the survival of penicillin-resistant bacteria, should that ever be an objective, but very little which assists in extermination. Yet some forms of penicillin-resistance arise by mutation, and genic recombinations among potentially-resistant species might well limit the usefulness of the newer penicillins, especially since resistance, once developed, usually extends to all available derivatives and even to cephalosporins. On the epidemiological side, there is no unified system or planned attempt to trace, register and probe resistance when it occurs, though the existence these days of international agencies and computers could easily expedite such investigation on an elastic and adaptable scale. This is a way of stating that the over-riding need is for team-work; the lesson of the past is that neither penicillin G nor the newer derivatives would have been identified or produced without team-work. It is just as likely that they will not be safeguarded without team-work in problems of clinical usage and resistance, though the team requires epidemiologists and geneticists as well as biochemists, microbiologists and clinicians. The team might find that laissez-faire is as good as anything but, if so, we should practise it advisedly and not speculatively.

REFERENCES

1 LURIA, S. E. AND DELBRUECK, M., *Genetics, 28* (1943) 491.
2 DEMEREC, M., *J. Bact., 36* (1948) 63.
3 LEDERBERG, J., *Genetics, 32* (1947) 505.
4 NEWCOMBE, H. B. AND NYHOLM, M. H., *Genetics, 35* (1950) 603.
5 HOTCHKISS, R. D., *Cold Spr. Harb. Symp. Quant. Biol., 16* (1951) 437.
6 ZINDER, N. D. AND LEDERBERG, J., *J. Bact., 64* (1952) 679.
7 MANTEN, A., *Bull. Wld Hlth. Org., 29* (1963) 387.
8 CAVALLE-SFORZA, L. L. AND LEDERBERG, J., *Genetics, 41* (1956) 367.
9 HINSHELWOOD, C. N., *The chemical kinetics of the bacterial cell*, Clarendon Press, Oxford, 1946.
10 POLLOCK, M. R., In DAVIES, R. AND GALE, E. F. (Eds.), *Adaptation in micro-organisms*, Cambridge University Press, 1953.
11 GERONIMUS, L. H. AND COHEN, S., *J. Bact., 73* (1957) 28.
12 HARMAN, SHIRLEY A. AND BALDWIN, J. N., *J. Bact., 87* (1964) 593.
13 MCDERMOTT, W., *Yale J. Biol. Med., 30* (1958) 257.
14 WATANABA, T. AND FUKASOWA, T., *J. Bact., 81* (1961) 669, 679.
15 POLLOCK, M. R. (1960) In MYRBÄCK, K., LARDY, H. AND BOYER, P. D. (Eds.), *The Enzymes*, (2nd ed.), Academic Press, New York, 1960.
16 FLOREY, H. W., *et al.*, *Antibiotics*, Vol. 2, Oxford University Press, 1949.
17 SNEATH, P. H. A., *J. gen. Microbiol., 13* (1955) 561.
18 POLLOCK, M. R., In *Resistance of bacteria to the penicillins*, Ciba Foundation Study Group No. 13, Churchill, London, 1962.
19 STEWART, G. T., *J. Hyg. (Lond.), 45* (1947) 282.
20 CITRI, N., *Biochim. Biophys. Acta, 27* (1961) 277.
21 POLLOCK, M. R., TORRIANI, A. M. AND TRIDGELL, E., *Biochem. J., 62* (1956) 387.
22 KOGUT, M., POLLOCK, M. R. AND TRIDGELL, E., *Biochem. J., 62* (1956) 391.
23 RICHMOND, M. H., *Biochem. J., 88* (1963) 452.
24 CROMPTON, B., JAGO, M., CRAWFORD, K., NEWTON, G. G. F. AND ABRAHAM, E. P., *Biochem. J., 83* (1962) 52.
25 STEWART, G. T., *Brit. med. J., II* (1960) 694.
26 STEINMAN, H. G., *Proc. Soc. exp. Biol. (N.Y.), 106* (1961) 227.
27 NOVICK, R. P., *Biochem. J., 83* (1962) 229.
28 HOLT, R. J. AND STEWART, G.T., *J. gen. Microbiol.*, (1964) (in the press).
29 BATCHELOR, F. R., CHAIN, E. B., RICHARDS, M. AND ROLINSON, G. N., *Proc. roy. Soc. B, 154* (1961) 522.
30 CLARIDGE, C. A., GOUREVITCH, A. AND LEIN, J., *Nature, 187* (1960) 237.
31 HOLT, R. J. AND STEWART, G. T., *Nature, 201* (1964) 824.
32 ENGLISH, A. R., MACBRIDE, T. J. AND HUANG, H. T., *Proc. Soc. exp. Biol. (N.Y.), 104* (1960) 50.
33 SMITH, J. T. AND HAMILTON-MILLER, J. M. T., *Nature, 197* (1963) 976.
34 KNOX, R. AND SMITH, J. T., *Lancet, ii* (1961) 520.

[35] BONDI, A. AND DIETZ, C. C., *Proc. Soc. exp. Biol. (N.Y.)*, *60* (1945) 55.
[36] KIRBY, W. M. M., *J. clin. Invest.*, *24* (1945) 165.
[37] BARBER, MARY, *J. Path. Bact.*, *59* (1947) 373.
[38] ROUNTREE, P. M. AND THOMSON, E. F., *Lancet, ii* (1949) 501.
[39] STEWART, G. T., *Brit. med. J.*, *I* (1961) 863.
[40] MUNCH-PETERSON, E. AND BOUNDY, C., *Bull. Wld Hlth. Org.*, *26* (1962) 241.
[41] SMITH, J. M. P. AND MARPLES, MARY J., *Nature*, *201* (1964) 844.
[42] JEVONS, M. PATRICIA, *Brit. med. J.*, *I* (1961) 124.
[43] STEWART, G. T. AND HOLT, R. J., *Brit. med. J.*, *I* (1963) 308.
[44] BECK, J. A. AND EVANS, I. L., *Brit. med. J.*, I (1963) 887.
[45] HARDING, J. W., *J. clin. Path.*, *16* (1963) 208.
[46] JEVONS, M. PATRICIA, COE, A. W. AND PARKER, M. T., *Lancet, i* (1963) 904.
[47] BOROWSKI, J., *Brit. med. J.*, *I* (1964) 983.
[48] RICHMOND, M. H., Personal communication, 1964.
[49] ERIKSEN, K. R., *Ugeskr. Laeg.*, *125* (1961) 1234.
[50] BARBER, MARY, In BRUMFITT, W. AND WILLIAMS, J. D. (Eds.), *Therapy with the new penicillins. Postgrad. med. J.*, *Suppl.*, *40*, 1964, p. 178.
[51] FARKAS-HIMSLEY, HANNAH AND SOEPRIHATIN, S. D., *Nature*, *202* (1964) 514.
[52] ELEK, S. D. AND FLEMING, P. C., *Lancet, ii* (1960) 569.
[53] GOLDFARB, SUSAN AND JAMES, G. C. W., *Brit. med. J.*, *I* (1963) 305.
[54] Report of a Committee, *Lancet, ii* (1961) 226.
[55] WILLCOX, R. R., In BRUMFITT, W. AND WILLIAMS, J. D. (Eds.), *Therapy with the new penicillins. Postgrad. med. J.*, *Suppl.*, *40*, 1964, p. 202.
[56] ALERGANT, C. D., In BRUMFITT, W. AND WILLIAMS, J. D. (Eds.), *Therapy with the new penicillins. Postgrad. med. J.*, *Suppl.*, *40*, 1964, p. 207.
[57] CHRISTIE, A. B., *Brit. med. J.*, *I* (1964) 1609.
[58] COLES, H. M. T., In BRUMFITT, W. AND WILLIAMS, J. D. (Eds.), *Therapy with new penicillins. Postgrad. med. J.*, *Suppl.*, *40*, 1964 (Discussion).
[59] POLLOCK, M. R., *Biochem. J.*, *66* (1957) 419.
[60] COOPER, P. D., *Bact. Rev.*, *20* (1956) 28.
[61] BARBER, M., *J. clin. Path.*, *14* (1961) 385.

Chapter 14

ALLERGY TO PENICILLINS

Hypersensitivity to penicillin was observed almost as soon as it became available for therapy. One of the first persons to be afflicted was a chemist engaged in research upon penicillin[1]. The earliest cases usually exhibited epidermal reactions[2] but other manifestations were soon noticed[3] after topical or parenteral administration of the drug[4] and attempts made, at first by giving small, incremental oral doses to desensitise patients[5]. From numerous other reports which then appeared, it became obvious that the causes and manifestations of penicillin allergy were multiple. Topical applications, leading to local reactions when penicillin was given subsequently by any route, were easily recognised and, by 1948, topical therapy was rightly regarded with disfavour. But reactions occurred also, if less frequently, in patients who had received the drug parenterally or sucked lozenges, often for trivial complaints which never merited penicillin therapy. Reviewing the incidence prior to 1950, Gilman[6] blamed many of the reactions on "the guilt of usage rather than of the substance". By 1963, the incidence in a survey made of 51000 beds in 95 hospitals in America was 59 anaphylactoid reactions, including 19 deaths; one patient had died after swallowing one tablet (100 or 200 mg) of an early oral penicillin, dibenzylethylenediamine penicillin G[7]. The incidence among nurses handling penicillin was often higher than among patients and many nurses were so highly sensitised that they had to abandon their profession[8].

In 1953, the Council on Pharmacy and Chemistry of the American Medical Association[9] drew attention to the prevalence of hypersensitivity. This action was prompted by the appearance of a new formulation of penicillin, penethamate hydroiodide, with different pharmacological properties and an affinity for pulmonary tissue. This proved to be not only toxic but highly allergenic; at the same time, it was noted that the procaine salt, formulated to delay absorption, introduced an added risk in that some subjects were sensitive to procaine by itself. The use of long-acting preparations (esters and oils) may also have increased the risk by providing a depot of sensitising antigen in the tissues.

References p. 171/172

Until this time, it had usually been assumed that sensitisation occurred as a result of previous exposure to some form of penicillin. The impression grew however that unmistakable anaphylaxis could occur in individuals who had never received the drug. Calvert and Smith[10] recorded a striking instance of this in a soldier who reacted first to a lozenge and then violently to an intramuscular injection. Reviewing the literature, these authors commented upon the seemingly high incidence in subjects with an allergic diathesis, especially in asthmatics, but many reactions occurred also in patients who had not been given, or who had not been told that they had been given, penicillin. They recommended, among other measures, that patients should be told that they had received penicillin, that physicians prescribing it should enquire if the patient had received it beforehand, and that injections should be given with a 45-second safety pause after the first fraction to permit immediate anaphylactic reactions to be detected.

At this stage, intradermal and scratch tests on the skin began to be widely practised to detect hypersensitivity but it soon became apparent that negative skin reactions, like negative histories, were not foolproof; in contrast, some patients reacted violently, even fatally, to skin tests and there was always a danger that further sensitisation could be caused by the test itself. Antihistamine drugs were therefore recommended[11] when a patient was known or thought to be sensitive; there was evidence that these were more effective when given intramuscularly before penicillin, or mixed with it. Some physicians devised schedules for active desensitisation on the principle of giving minute injections at one or more sites, increasing gradually on the lines established for pollen desensitisation. O'Driscoll[12] described a complex planned schedule in which a nurse was desensitised by 27 injections, at various sites, intradermally, subcutaneously and intramuscularly, under an antihistamine umbrella, in two weeks.

Penicillinase was also suggested[13] as a neutraliser in allergic reactions but this is unsatisfactory, not least because penicillinase, being a protein, is itself antigenic. It is usual therefore to use adrenaline or ephedrine[14] for controlling acute reactions, and there is justification for using antihistaminic agents (refs. 15, 16) for further suppression or prevention of the reaction, though the value of these drugs is held in question by some authorities.

The true incidence of hypersensitivity is extremely difficult to estimate, but the position has certainly been reached where penicillins rank as major causes of allergic reactions. In 1949, Keefer[17] estimated the incidence in subjects who had received penicillin as 3–5%. In 1963, Shelley[18] suggested that the figure might be as high as 10% in the United States. In countries where penicillin can be bought without prescription, the figure might be even higher[19] but in some other countries, including the United Kingdom, it is probably much lower. Even so, the manifestations of penicillin allergy (see p. 134) are so protean[20] that almost any reaction in any patient receiving the drug becomes suspicious: vasomotor changes, from faintness to collapse; anaphylactic shock, with oedema and urticaria, sometimes fatal; skin rashes, local or remote; convulsions[21]; agranulocytosis[22]; purpura and thrombocytopenia; Loeffler's syndrome with eosinophilia[18]; asthma. The most common reaction is pruritis and urticaria, ascribed to histamine release from mast cells in the skin[16]; in highly sensitised subjects, this release is more generalised, causing sneezing, pulmonary changes with dyspnoea, oedema, fall in blood pressure and shock. Eosinophilia and thrombocytopenia may occur during this. The degree of sensitisation can be extraordinarily high: deaths have been recorded[18,23] after skin tests with 10 units of penicillin G, and the writer knows of nurses who have exhibited unmistakable urticarial and vasomotor reactions merely by handling penicillins, in tablet form or in filling syringes.

In view of this unpredictable incidence, sometimes in subjects who have never received the drug, the question arises as to whether sensitisation to penicillin can arise from non-therapeutic preparations. It is known that the mould is commonly airborne—otherwise it might never have been discovered—and that many penicillia produce penicillin or closely related substances. The most obvious natural habitat of these moulds is decaying food, such as bread, cheese and fruit—the most productive strain, NRRL. 1951. B25, was isolated in 1941 from a rotten melon found in the Peoria market—which someone has to handle. An unexpected clue is offered by the recent finding in New Zealand[24] that hedgehogs are heavily infected by *T. mentagrophytes* which produces a penicillin-like substance in sufficient quantity to permit secondary infection only by penicillin-resistant staphylococci; possibly other rodents and man can be likewise infected. These possibilities, together with the fact that penicillin is often present in milk[25] make it very likely that sensitisation can arise and be provoked from various other sources[26-28]. The size of the problem is not confined to the unfortunate patients who exhibit hypersensitivity, though this is serious enough: in one recent estimate, deaths in the U.S.A. from anaphylaxis to penicillin may be as high as 300 in one year[29], while the incidence of lesser reactions is very much higher. Under these circumstances, any eruption or unexpected disturbance occurring during penicillin therapy tends to be ascribed to hypersensitivity, with the result that many patients who genuinely need the drug are denied its benefits.

References p. 171/172

This is undoubtedly the most confusing and perhaps the most urgent matter in penicillin therapy; no easy solution is in sight, but the problem is being discussed here and elsewhere in this book at some length so that some of the ecological and clinical factors may be kept in mind along with recent immunological work on the mechanism of hypersensitivity, for the wider use of the new penicillins may in some respects have increased the risk of provoking or incurring these reactions.

PRODUCTION OF ALLERGY IN EXPERIMENTAL ANIMALS

This is not so easy as it might seem. Benzyl penicillin and its analogues can be repeatedly injected and even applied topically without sensitisation necessarily occurring. A complicated programme of injections in oil–water emulsions has to be followed, on lines described by Chisholm et al.[30] in which rabbits are given several simultaneous injections, subcutaneously and intracutaneously; further subcutaneous injections are then given at weekly intervals. The animals are then bled and their sera tested for haemagglutinating power (q.v.) against homologous erythrocytes coated with penicillin. Guinea pigs can be sensitised by a similar method and tested for skin sensitivity after depilation.

Experimental allergy thus induced can be used to study antipenicillin antibodies[31], passive cutaneous anaphylaxis and Arthus phenomena pursuant to the study of the hypersensitive state. The technique has been invaluable in demonstrating differences in immunogenic potency of penicillins, especially when the haemagglutinin titre is measured. Nevertheless, it may exaggerate factors of lesser relevance in man; for instance, the haemagglutinin reaction may relate more to anaphylaxis and serum sickness[32] and may be negative in some subjects who exhibit only cutaneous hypersensitivity, while positive reactions have been recorded in patients who tolerate injections of penicillin[18]. It has been claimed[33] that macacque monkeys can be passively skin-sensitised and used for the diagnosis of human allergy.

MECHANISM OF HYPERSENSITIVITY TO PENICILLINS

It was at first assumed that penicillin combined with protein to form an antigenic complex, and that the various manifestations of hypersensitivity which followed applications or injections of penicillin were due to antibodies to this complex. This idea was supported by the fact that many of the earliest cases had been sensitised by topical applications of penicillin to infected skin, where local binding by protein in the exudate excited the process. It is true that, in subjects with this type of allergy, a local reaction at the original site often characterises any subsequent hypersensitivity, even when the drug is applied at a remote site or systemically. It is known also that many simple molecules serve as haptens to initiate antibody formation when protein-bound[34,35]. This only happens however when the molecule is reactive and forms stable protein conjugates *in vitro*[36]. Penicillins do not generally come into this category for, at neutral pH, they form mainly unstable conjugates with serum albumin which have not been shown to be immunogenic.

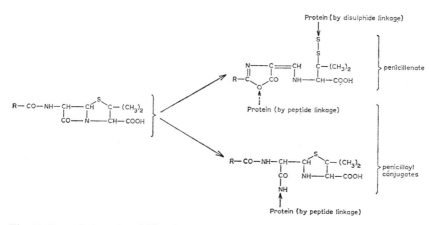

Fig. 11. Degradation of penicillins (R = side-chain) to form penicillenate and penicilloyl conjugates with proteins or amino acid complexes.

An alternative explanation has been offered by De Weck, Levine, Parker and others[37-39], who assumed that, since penicillin is relatively unstable, its degradation products might react with proteins, polypeptides and amino acids to form an antigenic substance. One of these products is penicillenic acid[40], which is formed quickly by most penicillins in solution, especially at an acid pH, though penicillin G forms it readily at pH 7.4. To form penicillenic acid, the thiazolidine ring of the penicillin nucleus is opened, leaving a free sulphydryl group which can link with proteins or polypeptides to form stable penicillenate conjugates; alternatively, the carbonyl group of the oxazolone group in penicillenic acid can react with amino groups (Fig. 11). Such conjugates would satisfy the theoretical requirements for antibody pro-

References p. 171/172

duction[41] and it has in fact been shown that they are antigenic to the rabbit and guinea pig[39]. At neutral pH, the second mechanism predominates; that is, formation of a penicilloyl conjugate by peptide linkage with amino groups. Specific antibodies can be demonstrated as precipitins or haemagglutinins, and hypersensitivity by passive cutaneous anaphylaxis and Arthus reactions in animals, and by the wheal-and-erythema reaction in man after passive transfer (Prausnitz–Küstner test). These reactions are inhibited by the corresponding haptens of penicilloyl or penicillenate structure, between which there is no cross-reaction.

The experimental evidence for this hypothesis is very strong. Not only do animals injected with these conjugates exhibit hypersensitivity; if haemagglutination titres against penicillin-coated red cells be taken as an index, the immunogenic power of a given penicillin is closely proportional to its rate of degradation to penicillenic acid. Thus, according to De Weck, penicillin G which degrades quickly at pH 7.4 is more immunogenic than methicillin which degrades more slowly; phenethicillin, which scarcely degrades, is hypo-immunogenic.

There are however some anomalies even in the experimental evidence. De Weck[42] maintains that haemolysis, which occurs when cells are coated by the penicillin, is a further reflection of the sensitising potential of the penicillin; whereas in fact penicillin G, which provokes high agglutinin titres, causes minimal haemolysis, but phenethicillin and propicillin[43], which scarcely raise the haemagglutinin titre and do not degrade readily, produce active haemolysins.

If these experimental results are related to clinical hypersensitivity, it is necessary to assume that a penicilloyl or other degradation product conjugates with protein when penicillin is first introduced into the body to act as a specific antigen, initiating antibody formation. How then does a subsequent injection of penicillin, or exposure to it, elicit hypersensitivity? According to immunological theory, the provocative dose must also be conjugated in such a way that the organic determinant (penicillin) is multivalent, i.e. is present at more than one site on the protein molecule[44]. In practice[38], benzyl penicillenic acid conjugates with γ-globulin at pH 7.5 and penicilloyl proteins are able to evoke cutaneous responses in a high proportion of subjects known to be allergic to penicillin[45], whereas unconjugated degradation products or pure penicillin often fail to produce a reaction; this may be due to these substances acting as univalent inhibitors of the reaction by combining with the antipenicilloyl antibody[46]. This would appear to explain the anomalies of intradermal or scratch tests, for it is certainly common experience that subjects with a proved history of hypersensitivity often fail to react to skin tests with penicillins, though it is also known that some such subjects will react strongly to doses as small as 0.01 μg of freshly-prepared penicillin G or even to the mere handling of the drug. If the penicilloyl-hapten theory is correct, conjugation must occur very rapidly, perhaps per-cutaneously, in these subjects and might well provoke release of histamine and further sensitisation. To obviate this risk, Parker and his colleagues[47] treated penicillenic acid with a polymer of lysine to obtain a product of lower molecular weight than the protein conjugate, but containing by lysine-bonding multiple penicilloyl groups (penicilloyl polylysine). This proved to be less immunogenic experimentally than penicilloyl protein but was almost equally effective in evoking skin reactions in allergic patients attending a venereal disease clinic in St. Louis. The reactions were inhibited by the homologous univalent hapten, ε-penicilloylaminocaproate. No sensitisation attributable to the penicilloyl polylysine was observed, nor were there any severe reactions to the test.

In these studies, and in similar tests with penicilloyl polylysines conducted in Switzerland[41], the incidence of positive skin reactions in persons with a history of penicillin allergy is as high as 75–81 %. In studies conducted elsewhere the figure is lower[46], about 30 %. Until this anomaly is explained by further work, it must be concluded that the penicilloyl polylysines, while more reliable as skin-test reagents than unmodified penicillins, cannot be guaranteed to give a reaction in all sensitised subjects. The possibility remains that the most highly-sensitised subjects, liable to immediate anaphylactic reactions, can always be detected by skin tests; in which case the penicilloyl polylysines should now be used instead of pure penicillins or protein conjugates as test substances, since they are less likely to cause further sensitisation or severe reactions.

The exact nature of the antigenic determinant or determinants also awaits further elucidation. According to Parker and Thiel[48], the polylysines prepared from penicillin G and penicillenic acid are equally potent in skin tests, so that in their opinion the penicilloyl group is the primary antigenic determinant. In rabbits, protein conjugates formed from penicillenic acid and penicilloyl groups are immunogenic but antibodies formed against the penicilloyl groups prevail over those formed from penicillenate[48] which accords with the pattern of conjugation at neutral pH. It would appear likely therefore that penicilloyl structures are major antigenic determinants. This may not account for all reactions, however, for it is known that the immunogenicity of a given penicillin is related to the extent of its degradation to penicillenic acid; penicillenate structures and other haptenic groups may therefore

References p. 171/172

play a part, including possibly the side-chain. In the case of penicillin G, Levine and Ovary[49] consider that the N-(D-α-benzylpenicilloyl) group, formed by lysine bonding, is the antigenic determinant; allergy is antibody-dependent and can be inhibited by the homologous N-(α-D-penicilloyl) amines, acting as univalent haptens. In other respects, the role of the side-chain is uncertain and the evidence conflicting. As judged by their immunogenic powers in rabbits, there are considerable differences between, for instance, phenethicillin and penicillin G, yet both can act as sensitising agents on red cells, or as allergens in cutaneous tests. If penicillenate structures are involved in these reactions, phenethicillin should be almost inert, as should 6-APA itself. On quantitative assessment, these substances are less active in all respects than penicillin G and methicillin, but they are active and, if the degradation theory is correct, it is hard to believe that penicillenic acid is not a factor in eliciting a reaction when penicillin is injected in solution. Yet the more consistent reactivity and higher specificity[48] of the penicilloyl polylysines in cutaneous tests seem to exclude the penicillenates as major allergens. This recalls the original idea that the intact penicillin molecule somehow forms stable conjugates with proteins when injected; direct conjugation with γ-globulin is said to enhance skin-reactivity in subjects liable to the urticarial-serum sickness type of hypersensitivity[50]. If direct linkage is the explanation of this, the locus could be one of several: the antigenicity and allergenicity of 6-APA suggest the possibility of linkage to the free amino group; alternatively, in some of the derivatives, linkage might occur to the free amino groups of proteins.

There is clearly a relationship of some kind between these experimental results and clinical hypersensitivity but it is difficult to prove or disprove this directly. If penicilloyl conjugates (polylysines) are used intradermally or by scratch test in human subjects with a history of hypersensitivity to penicillin, a high proportion (over 80% according to De Weck) exhibit an immediate wheal-and-erythema response whereas, with penicillin G as test substance, the proportion is certainly much lower. It is common experience that subjects with a suggestive history of hypersensitivity may fail to react to a skin test with penicillin G, but it is also true that some such subjects react to amounts as small as 0.01 μg. According to Parker and Thiel, the polylysines prepared from penicillin G and penicillenic acid are equally potent in eliciting positive reactions in sensitised subjects so that, in their opinion, the penicilloyl group is the primary antigenic determinant; preparations free from penicillenates and other degradation intermediates are active but the benzyl side-chain may be a potent secondary factor since polylysines prepared (at alkaline pH) from this are more reactive than those made with other penicillins. Levine[38] found that benzyl penicillenic acid conjugated with γ-globulin at pH 7.5 and suggested that this could react with antibody in sensitised subjects.

There is therefore good evidence that the degradation products of penicillins are involved in some or all of the manifestations of allergy, chiefly through the formation of penicilloyl conjugates. It is also claimed that these conjugates may be more useful than the parent penicillins for the detection of allergy by skin tests, partly because they may give a higher incidence of true positive reactions and partly because they never evoke severe or generalised reactions or aggravate hypersensitivity, as may occur with unconjugated penicillin. Further evidence must accrue before this possibility is accepted; there is an inconsistency in the suggestion that the conjugates are harmful as systemic antigens and harmless as skin antigens. Irrespectively of the hypothesis, however, the conjugates offer promise as diagnostic reagents. This was realised, on empirical grounds, before the work of De Weck, Parker and others, since the use of pure penicillin G as a skin test reagent undoubtedly fails to detect many cases of severe hypersensitivity[19]. The experimental techniques devised to explore the problem also offer opportunities for testing new penicillins less subject to degradation.

Meanwhile, the problem of overcoming hypersensitivity awaits solution. All penicillins so far prepared for therapy are cross-allergenic. This was shown in 1950 by Risman and Boger[51] when butylthiomethyl penicillin and allylmercaptomethyl penicillin were prepared. Later, when new derivatives of 6-APA were prepared, allergic reactions were also noted and it was found (ref. 52) that complete cross-allergenicity existed between the therapeutic forms of penicillin and also the 6-APA nucleus itself, though the presence in this of traces of benzyl penicillin is difficult to exclude. There are, however, differences in the degree of allergenicity demonstrable to the various penicillins. This suggests that the side-chain may have some influence in modifying allergenicity but, with the possible exception of 4-carboxy-n-butyl, about which evidence is conflicting[53-55], no side-chain has yet been described which abolishes cross-allergenicity, as tested by a variety of techniques[18,52,56-58]. The cephalosporanic acid nucleus, however, differing only in the replacement of the penicillin thiazolidine ring by a dihydrothiazine ring (Chapter 16), together with its benzyl and other derivatives, is not cross-allergenic in human subjects[52] which suggests that the major determinant in this respect is in or linked to the thiazolidine part of 6-APA, or to the lactam ring.

The present state of knowledge about hypersensitivity is an incomplete jigsaw of experimental chemical and clinical bits of data. The overall pattern is beginning to emerge but the interrelationships of some of the bits is still obscure. Immunogenic power in a given penicillin has to be assessed experimentally in animals, usually by the production of haemagglutinating antibodies. Similar antibodies can be found in the sera of some patients with allergy to penicillin[59] but not consistently. Several critical studies have shown discrepancies between serological results and allergic manifestations[60-62]. In a recent re-examination of this problem, Van Arsdel and his colleagues[32] found that the haemagglutinin test could be made more sensitive and more specific by diluting the coated red cells in serum from the same donor. Thus tested, 69% of patients with known anaphylaxis or angioedema, and 50% of those with serum sickness after penicillin, had haemagglutinating antibodies. The test was less frequently positive (20%) in patients with urticarial reactions and was uniformly negative in those with miscellaneous rashes. Positive skin tests were rare and occurred only in severe anaphylactic subjects, so that they were "closely allied with acute life-threatening reactions". Van Arsdel's findings are unconfirmed as yet, and they contradict many previous impressions. One explanation of this may lie again in the need for conjugation of penicilloyl groups in coating the red cells; this occurs more effectively at alkaline pH, cells so treated agglutinate to higher titres, and the reaction can be inhibited by penicillin G or by penicilloyl ε-aminocaproate, which is a thousand times more active[63] in this respect. It is claimed also[46] that the ^{131}I-labelled penicilloyl antigen in the γ-globulin fractions of sera from allergic patients can be easily precipitated by rabbit antihuman globulin sera and that this also is reduced by the univalent ε-aminocaproate hapten. It is possible therefore that the same type of γ-globulin antibody in the 7-S and 19-S fractions is being produced in experimental rabbits as in human subjects who have received penicillin G[64]. The question remains as to whether or not this antibody is formed only as an allergic process. Even in Van Arsdel's study, falsely-positive haemagglutinating antibodies were found in sera from subjects who had no evidence of specific allergy and in one sample of cord blood. Nevertheless, there can be little doubt that the role of the penicilloyl conjugates as allergens and as antigens is established, and that these substances are concerned in human serological responses to penicillin.

Evidence cited earlier in this chapter points to other mechanisms besides penicilloyl conjugation being involved in the cutaneous reaction. The same may be true of the allergic state generally, for it is extremely unlikely that manifestations as diverse as those observed in penicillin hypersensitivity have one collective biochemical explanation. A further set of variables is introduced by the differing structures and formulations of the penicillins themselves. A substance such as penicillin G, which is rapidly excreted and forms no known residual metabolites in tissue, obviously has a limited sensitising potential; whereas long-acting compounds can behave very differently: it is estimated that a single injection of benzathine penicillin induces cutaneous sensitivity to penicilloyl polylysine in 5–10% of subjects[46] and it is likely that depot preparations used for dental purposes do likewise[65].

Hypersensitivity in its dramatic diversity is undoubtedly the only serious hazard in therapy with the penicillins. If it cannot be prevented, it can at least be minimised by rational application of the considerable body of knowledge which has now accumulated. The following practical measures are certainly justified:

(1) Topical applications to the skin and mucous membranes should be avoided.

(2) Injections into closed cavities such as empyemas should be given only when systemic treatment fails to produce therapeutic concentrations in these sites, and where alternative agents cannot be employed. Joint cavities and the subarachnoid space may be exceptions to this rule.

(3) Lozenges and nasal drops should not be used. Ocular, dental and aural formulations should be viewed with caution.

(4) For parenteral use the penicillins should be obtained as dry crystals or powders in the pure state, and dissolved in water buffered to an optimal pH immediately before injection.

(5) Caution should be exercised in the use of long-acting and depot formulations.

(6) The shelf-life of existing therapeutic preparations should be assessed in terms of degradation products as well as antibacterial activity.

(7) Patients for whom penicillin is prescribed should as far as practicable be informed of this fact. This is especially important when further courses of any penicillin are likely to be required, or when long-acting or depot formulations are used. Long-term prescriptions should not be issued without opportunity for review, and any unused tablets or ampoules should be returned or discarded.

(8) Self-medication by nurses, medical auxiliaries, pharmaceutical workers and others should be discouraged.

(9) Before any penicillin is prescribed or administered, the patient (or parents or relatives) should be asked if he has any knowledge of having received it before.

(10) Patients with a history or any manifestation suggestive of penicillin

allergy should be skin-tested with penicilloyl polylysine. If this is positive, penicillin should not normally be used; if negative, the drug may be given under careful surveillance with a 45-second safety pause if it is injected. Additional tests for hypersensitivity, such as the haemagglutination reaction and the basophil degranulation test, may help to identify hypersensitive subjects who react negatively to skin tests.

(*11*) Highly sensitised subjects should be desensitised (see p. 160), especially if working in a hospital or clinic.

(*12*) If a penicillin has to be administered for over-riding therapeutic reasons to a hypersensitive subject, a suitable and acceptable antihistamine drug should be given concurrently. There is no doubt that some hypersensitive patients can be treated successfully in this way and, if a penicillin must be employed (*e.g.* for osteomyelitis or septicaemia), there is every justification for following this procedure. Some authorities[66] doubt the value of prophylactic antihistamines and, in any event, it is wise to have adrenaline and ephedrine readily available also throughout such therapy.

(*13*) All available therapeutic penicillins are cross-allergenic but probably in widely-differing degrees. Severe anaphylactic reactions have been attributable mainly to penicillins G and V which may therefore become penicillins of second choice where allergy is suspected.

(*14*) Asthmatics and other patients with allergic diatheses appear to be much more likely than others to become sensitised to penicillins. If these drugs are employed, tests for sensitivity should be performed at frequent intervals, using the penicilloyl polylysines for skin tests to avoid further sensitisation.

If these safeguards are observed, penicillins can continue to be used widely but not complacently. Some existing, well-established therapeutic habits may require alteration, and research might well be directed towards the production of penicillins of lower allergenicity or to the use of antagonists such as the univalent haptens. If substances of this kind prove to be non-toxic, they might be given with penicillins to lessen their antigenicity or allergenicity in cases at risk, or they might assist in certain stages of the desensitisation process. Alternatively, it is conceivable that penicillins can be produced which do not degrade into substances with potential antigenicity. The known antigenicity[30] and cross-allergenicity of 6-APA is an obstacle in this respect and it may be more promising to consider the possibility of nuclear modification. For immediate purposes, the only β-lactam antibiotics with comparable antibacterial properties are certain cephalosporins, *i.e.* derivatives of 7-aminocephalosporanic acid and, in them, the difference in nuclear structure seems to abolish cross-allergenicity (Table XVII).

TABLE XVII

CROSS-ALLERGENICITY TO β-LACTAM ANTIBIOTICS
(Intradermal tests in individuals with cutaneous hypersensitivity)

Ring	Side-chain	Number sensitive Number tested
6-APA	NIL	7/10
(penicillins)	benzyl (Penicillin G)	10/10
	p-amino	2/2
	α-amino (Ampicillin)	6/6
	dimethoxy (Methicillin)	9/10
	chlorphenyl isoxazolyl (Cloxacillin)	2/2
	α-aminoadipyl (Penicillin N)	3/3
7-ACA	NIL	0/1
(cephalosporins)	benzyl	0/4
	thioenyl (Cephalothin)	0/1
	(Cephaloridine)	0/5
	α-aminoadipyl (Cephalosporin C)	0/5

REFERENCES

1 SILVERS, S. H., *Arch. Derm.-Syph. (N.Y.)*, 50 (1944) 328.
2 PYLE, H. D. AND RATTNER, H., *J. Amer. med. Assoc.*, 125 (1944) 903.
3 CRIEP, L. H., *J. Amer. med. Assoc.*, 126 (1944) 429.
4 WILENSKY, A. O., *J. Amer. med. Assoc.*, 131 (1946) 1384.
5 O'DONOVAN, W. J. AND KLORFAJN, I., *Lancet, ii* (1946) 444.
6 GILMAN, R. L., *U.S. armed Forces med., J.* 1 (1950) 1155.
7 WELCH, H., LEWIS, C. N., KERLAN, I. AND PUTNAM, L. A., *Antibiot. Chemotherap.*, 3 (1953) 89.
8 Ministry of Health, special report, 1953.
9 *J. Amer. med. Assoc.*, 151 (1953) 1105.
10 CALVERT, R. J. AND SMITH, E., *Brit. med. J.*, II (1955) 302.
11 BECK, C. A., *J. Amer. med. Assoc.*, 153 (1953) 1170.
12 O'DRISCOLL, B. J., *Brit. med. J.*, II (1955) 473.
13 BECKER, R. M., *Practitioner*, 184 (1958) 447.
14 LOWELL, F. C., *New Eng. J. Med.*, 268 (1963) 218.
15 MATHEWS, K. P., HEMPHILL, F. M., LOVALL, R. G., FORSYTHE, W. E. AND SHELDON, J. M., *J. Allergy*, 27 (1956) 1.
16 KELLER, R., *Experientia*, 18 (1962) 286.
17 KEEFER, C. S., In IRVING G. W. AND HERRICK, H. T. (Eds.), *Antibiotics*, Chem. Pub. Co., Brooklyn, 1949.
18 SHELLEY, W. B., *J. Amer. med. Assoc.*, 184 (1963) 171.
19 IDSÖE, E. AND WANG, K. Y., *Bull. Wld Hlth Org.*, 18 (1958) 323.
20 BLANTON, W. B. AND BLANTON, F. M., *J. Allergy*, 24 (1953) 405.
21 HUMPHRIES, S. O., *Lancet, i* (1963) 115.
22 SIGAL, E. S., *Kazan Med. Zh.*, 1 (1963) 59 (Russian).
23 MOUGAR, J. L. AND SCHILD, H. O., *Physiol. Rev.*, 42, (1962) 226.

172   ALLERGY TO PENICILLINS

24 SMITH, J. M. P. AND MARPLES, MARY J., *Nature*, 201 (1964) 844.
25 *Antibiotics in milk in Great Britain*, Report of the Milk Hygiene Subcommittee, London, H.M.S.O., 1963.
26 WELCH, H., *Am. J. Pub. Health*, 47 (1957) 701.
27 SIEGEL, B. B., *Bull. Wld Hlth Org.*, 21 (1959) 703.
28 BORRIE, P. AND BARRETT, J., *Brit. med. J.*, II (1961) 1267.
29 FEINBERG, S. M., *J. Amer. med. Assoc.*, 178 (1961) 815.
30 CHISHOLM, D. R., ENGLISH, A. R. AND MACLEAN. N. A., *J. Allergy*, 32 (1961) 333.
31 DE WECK, A. L., *Arch. Allergy*, 21 (1962) 20.
32 VAN ARSDEL, P. P., O'ROURKE, T. K., HOSAN, J. D. AND KUMASAKIA, Y., *J. Amer. med. Assoc.*, 185 (1953) 584.
33 LAYTON, L. L., SEE, S. AND DEEDS, F., *Proc. Soc. exp. Biol. (N.Y.)*, 108 (1961) 623.
34 LANDSTEINER, K., *The specificity of serological reactions*, Harvard Univerisity Press, Cambridge, (Mass), 1945, p. 200.
35 GELL, P. G. H., HARRINGTON, C. R. AND MICHEL, R., *Brit. J. exp. Path.*, 27 (1946) 267.
36 EISEN, H. N., In LAWRENCE, H.S. (Ed.), *Cellular and humoral aspects of the hypersensitive states*, Harper–Hoeber, New York, 1959.
37 DE WECK, A. L. AND EISEN, H. N., *J. exp. Med.*, 112 (1960) 1227.
38 LEVINE, B. B., *Arch. Biochem. Biophys.*, 93 (1961) 50.
39 PARKER, C. W., DE WECK, A. L., KERN, M. AND EISEN, H. N., *J. exp. Med.*, 115 (1962) 803.
40 CARPENTER, F. H., TURNER, R. A. AND DU VIGNEAUD, V., *J. biol. Chem.*, 176 (1948) 893.
41 DE WECK, A. L., *Int. Arch. Allergy*, 22 (1963) 245.
42 DE WECK, A. L., *Int. Arch. Allergy*, 21 (1962) 20, 38.
43 FEINBERG, J. G., Personal communication, 1964.
44 CAMPBELL, D. H. AND MCCASLAND, G. E., *J. Immunol.*, 49 (1944) 315.
45 LEVINE, B. B., *J. exp. Med.*, 114 (1961) 875.
46 PARKER, C. W., *Amer. J. Med.*, 34 (1963) 747.
47 PARKER, C. W., SHAPIRO, J., KERN, M. AND EISEN, H. N., *J. exp. Med.*, 115 (1962) 821.
48 PARKER, C. W. AND THIEL, J. A., *J. lab. clin. Med.*, 62 (1963) 482.
49 LEVINE, B. B. AND OVARY, Z., *J. exp. Med.*, 114 (1961) 875.
50 RAJKA, G. AND VINEZE, ELIZABETH, *Ann. Allergy*, 16 (1958) 291.
51 RISMAN, G. AND BOGER, W. P., *J. Allergy*, 21 (1950) 425.
52 STEWART, G. T., *Lancet*, i (1962) 509.
53 FLOREY, H. W., *Ann. int. Med.*, 43 (1955) 480.
54 BALLIO, A., *Nature*, 185 (1960) 97.
55 LEY, A. B., HARRIS, JEAN P., BRINKLEY, MARY, LILES, B., JACK, J. A. AND CAHAN, A., *Science*, 127 (1958) 1118.
56 CRIEP, L. H. AND FRIEDMAN, H., *New Eng. med. J.*, 263 (1960) 891.
57 EPP, Marguerite, *Science*, 130 (1959) 1472.
58 DE WECK, A. L., *Int. Arch. Allergy*, 21 (1962) 38.
59 LEY, A. B., *Science*, 127 (1958) 1118.
60 HEGGIE, A. D., *New Eng. J. Med.*, 262 (1960) 1160.
61 WATSON, K. C., JOUBERT, S. M. AND BENNETT, M. A. E., *Immunology*, 3 (1960) 1.
62 WATSON, K. C., JOUBERT, S. M. AND BENNETT, M. A. E., *Immunology*, 4 (1961) 193.
63 FUDENBERG, H. S. AND GERMAN, J. L., *Blood*, 15 (1960) 683.
64 WATSON, K. C., *Immunology*, 7 (1964) 97.
65 HARLEY, H. J., *Arch. Derm. (Chic.)*, 87 (1963) 387.
66 *Brit. med. J.*, II (1963) 1643, Today's Drugs.

Chapter 15

EPIDEMIOLOGICAL IMPACT

To anyone versed in the traditional intractability of severe, systemic pyoge-
ic infection, the clinical impact of penicillin G began to be obvious almost
overnight and was taken for granted by 1945. In this sense, history repeated
itself in 1960 when methicillin and its analogues restored the balance of
power against penicillin-resistant staphylococci. Nevertheless, important as
they are as clinical problems, the pyogenic infections play a relatively unimportant role in statistics of morbidity and mortality. The epidemiological
impact of the penicillins—as of most therapeutic substances—is therefore
comparatively slight if measured in terms of the incidence and mortality of
the major groups of diseases shown in national and international statistics.
This does not lessen their importance in the amelioration of infections and
even the vital statistics are not entirely unaffected if the following diseases are
considered:

Streptococcal infections

From an epidemiological viewpoint, the only streptococci which are important are those of group A which cause communicable infections such as
sore throat, impetigo, scarlet fever, puerperal sepsis and, secondarily, rheumatic fever, otitis media and glomerulonephritis. All of those diseases were
well-recognized in the thirties and earlier as major problems especially in
communities like schools, barracks and maternity hospitals. To a limited
extent, and notably in puerperal sepsis, the sulphonamides began to control
these infections from 1937 onward, but it is common knowledge—clinically
and epidemiologically—that the real fall in incidence was most noticeable
about 1945. There can be little doubt that penicillin played a part in this
probably, in the first place, by the rapid cure of simple throat infections
which formed by far the largest pool of streptococci in the community. It is
logical to deduce, even if there is no exact proof, that scarlet fever and the
other forms of infection which spread traditionally in the wake of strepto-

References p. 182/184

coccal sore throat were thereby also diminished, almost to the point of extinction in some communities. Early studies[1] showed that streptococci were eliminated in a few days from most cases of sore throat and scarlet fever; aural surgeons were commenting by 1946 on the decline of mastoiditis to the point of rarity[2,3]; and there was no doubt about the efficacy of penicillin in the prophylaxis of rheumatic fever (p. 31). These and other changes occurred before any other antibiotic with comparable activity appeared. Improvements in hygiene and welfare of the community undoubtedly played a part but cannot have diminished the infectivity of the organism, which remained prevalent.

The use of penicillin in these infections is now so habitual that figures for untreated cases are hard to find. An indication of the present position in rheumatic fever is given, however, by Stollerman and his colleagues[4] who studied recurrences of acute rheumatism in 385 patients who were not receiving penicillin prophylaxis. Seventy-eight per cent of these patients developed asymptomatic streptococcal infections which were not treated; of these 10% showed rheumatic recurrences. This figure (in adult and adolescent subjects) is lower than that of recurrence in childhood but it emphasizes the importance of prophylaxis[5,6] for, even when infection was symptomatic and therefore identifiable for treatment, the recurrence rate (11.7%) was not much higher.

It is doubtful if the newer penicillins offer any improvement over penicillin G in these infections; none is as active *in vitro* and, in therapy, penicillin G is so effective that it is rarely justifiable to contemplate the use of another drug, except in the presence of allergy or of another penicillin-resistant organism, for there are no reports of penicillin-resistance in group A streptococci. The latest authoritative view of chemoprophylaxis[7] recommends 1–2 mega units of benzathine penicillin monthly or 200,000 units of potassium penicillin G orally on an empty stomach. It is probably beneficial to continue this regime indefinitely in all subjects below 18 years of age who have had rheumatic heart disease and in all those above 18 years who have evidence of a rheumatic lesion even if it is inactive. In penicillin-sensitive subjects (and a measurable proportion will be sensitised if benzathine penicillin is used) sulphadiazine (1 g daily) is recommended as an alternative. The role of the acid-stable penicillins is questionable though cloxacillin or dicloxacillin[8] are eligible for use if penicillinase-forming staphylococci are present or acquired during the prophylactic regime.

Pneumococcal infection

Lobar pneumonia, in which the pneumococcus is usually the chief identifiable pathogen, was named by Osler (quoting John Bunyan) "Captain of the men of death"[9]. In the pre-chemotherapy era it predominated in mortality registrations at the extremes of age; even at intermediate ages, its mortality was by no means negligible. Serotherapy and sulphonamides played their part in reducing this mortality, but, again, the real decline came after 1945 when it became clear that, in the absence of organic complications, pneumococcal pneumonia was curable by penicillin so rapidly that in the words of one author[10] the disease met its Waterloo and the classical clinical picture became a rarity. The epidemiological consequences of this part of the therapeutic revolution were, however, complex: the reduction in incidence and morbidity of pneumococcal pneumonia in the elderly borrowed an interval of longevity which permitted degenerative and neoplastic diseases to increase and, in their turn, to create a predisposition to other diseases of debility, including pneumonia. In younger subjects, the reduction in pneumococcal infection left a zymotic vacuum which began to be replaced[11-14], though incompletely as yet, by other infective agents, including viruses and mycoplasma[15,16] which were and are less susceptible to chemotherapy[17]. The new penicillins are less active than penicillin G against the pneumococcus and appear to be generally ineffective against its pathogenic successors in pulmonary infection. The only exception is ampicillin which controls some forms of gram-negative pneumonia and holds a hint of activity against the virus of pneumonitis (Chapter 6).

Gonococcal infection

In the words of a sailor treated by the writer in 1944, penicillin reduced gonorrhoea to something "Less than a cold in the head". The clinical effect[18] even of a single injection[19] was certainly miraculous though it was perhaps the first miracle to confer an immediate and obvious benefit upon Sin. Possibly for this reason, the epidemiological sequelae to the introduction of penicillin therapy and prophylaxis left much to be desired: the incidence of gonorrhoea did not always decrease, especially among service personnel, and it was not long before drug-resistance began to occur[20,21], despite the high susceptibility of the organism.

At present, drug-resistance is of the order of 10- to 100-fold, yielding mutants inhibited by 0.125–1.0 μg/ml of penicillin G in about 15% of pa-

References p. 182/184

tients[22]. These mutants are resistant also to other forms of penicillin, including ampicillin, but they are still relatively sensitive to penicillin G in comparison with other drugs, so there is as yet no reason for any major departure from penicillin therapy[23]. The treatment introduced in 1948 with procaine penicillin G in oil with 2% aluminum monostearate (PAM) is still regarded as satisfactory for standard therapy. If the patient is hypersensitive to penicillin, tetracycline or dimethylchlortetracycline can be substituted[24]. Some cases resist therapy because of mixed infections with *Mimeae*[25] or other organisms, in which event amphotericin B or other drugs may be required as adjuvants. In a few refractory cases ampicillin has been found useful[26,27], but this may be because of its greater activity against other organisms causing secondary infection rather than to greater activity against the gonococcus. Recent evidence[23] suggests that an increase in resistant organisms is creating a problem in carriers and cases with residual infection. If this is so, an increase in the incidence of gonorrhoea would seem inevitable and it is doubtful if chemotherapy can do much to stop it unless vigorous social and educational programmes are executed concomitantly[28]. In the long run, a cold in the head might once again be the lesser evil.

Syphilis

The treatment of this disease with penicillin was slower in being evaluated owing to the need for a long clinical and serological follow-up. From 1943 onward, various courses were tried, usually consisting of one or more daily injections of the soluble sodium or potassium salts of penicillin G in water, arachis oil or beeswax, given 8–14 days in early primary infections, longer in late primary and secondary cases. The immediate clinical effects of even a few injections were impressive but it was soon found that intensive treatment was required to prevent relapses. The essential point is that a serum or plasma level of at least 0.03 units per ml must be maintained continuously for 10 days. If this is done, the cure rate is likely to be 95% or higher[29] in cases diagnosed early by direct recognition of *Treponema pallidum* in the primary lesion or by serology which should include nowadays a complement-fixation test performed with the Reiter treponemal antigen[30]. The formulation of procaine penicillin G in oil with aluminum monostearate (PAM) led to the introduction of a very effective one-shot treatment which was used from 1949 onward and played a considerable part in lowering the infectivity of cases seen haphazardly in seaports or amid mobile populations. The incidence of syphilis therefore fell to such an extent that it was described in 1958 as a "Dying disease"[31]. Since then there has been a recrudescence[28] amounting in 1962 to as much as 7% increase on the 1961 figures and, in 1963, even more[32] though this may be partly due to more thorough notification of early cases. The increase, which is international, is largely accounted for by infection of young people below 24 years of age or even in their teens.*

In these new circumstances, the epidemiological consequences of one-shot penicillin therapy are dubious. Education and contact-tracing are as essential in the control of venereal disease as is the drug, and this cannot be done if treatment appears to be casual or is too brief. The best treatment, according to the U.S. Public Health Service[33], is 4.8 mega units of aqueous procaine penicillin G given in 8 daily injections; King[23,29] suggests a slightly higher dosage (6 mega units in 10 days) and, in all except the earliest cases, it is essential that a higher dosage schedule of 6–9 mega units be employed. The long-acting depot preparations (PAM, benzathine penicillin) should be reserved for itinerant patients in whom, as a compromise, an initial injection of, say, 2.4 mega units (2.4 g) of PAM can be followed by two injections, each of 1.2 mega units at 3-day intervals. The initial dose will render all defaulting patients non-infective, and will cure a proportion. The U.S. Public Health Service recommends 4.8–9.6 mega units according to the stage of the infection.

No drug approaches penicillin G in the therapy of syphilis and, in primary and secondary cases, this is the only specific therapy required. In some tertiary or latent cases, and in neurosyphilis, bismuth is still used but arsenotherapy has been mostly abandoned. In infants with congenital syphilis, the total dosage of penicillin G is 200,000 units per lb. body-weight, equivalent in a $7\frac{1}{2}$ lb. baby to a daily dose of 150,000 units of procaine penicillin intramuscularly for 10 days. The new penicillins are less active than penicillin G against *Treponema pallidum*. Drug-resistance does not occur. If a patient is hypersensitive to penicillin, tetracycline or oxytetracycline are the preferred alternatives in a total dosage of 30–50 g, orally, over 10–15 days. Other antibiotics, including erythromycin and carbomycin are also active against the spirochaete[34] but all of them fall far short of penicillin G in efficacy.

Venereal disease is an international problem and it is essential that some uniformity be observed with regard to the formulation and activity of the penicillins used and also the procedure in clinics. The reports of expert committees of the World Health Organization[35] show that different preparations

* According to The New York Times (December 13, 1964) the increase in persons under 20 between 1956 and 1963 is over 200%. In some cities the figures for 1964 suggest that the disease is now epidemic in scale.

References p. 182/184

of PAM vary considerably and that surveillance and treatment of contacts, vital in the control of the disease, are omitted in a majority or special clinics in respresentative communities. The same conditions, and criticisms, apply to yaws.

With existing knowledge and available techniques properly applied, syphilis can be cured and prevented from spreading by the use of penicillin. Routine serology of pregnant women, with treatment of cases so detected, leads to prevention of congenital syphilis in at least 95 % of cases[36]. This is perhaps the most striking example of successful chemoprophylaxis in medicine.

Meningococcal infection

Penicillin G and ampicillin are effective therapeutically in this condition but not necessarily more so than sulphadiazine which has been for many years the standard treatment in many important centres for cases and universally, for carriers. Recent work by Feldman[37] and others[38] shows a clear trend toward increasing sulphonamide-resistance in meningococci, however, At the time of writing, it seems that about 20 % of strains isolated from civilian and military sources in the U.S.A. fall into this category. At this prevalence, prophylaxis by sulphadiazine ceases to be practicable and expectant therapy becomes hazardous. Penicillins G and V have not been found useful in clearing carriers but no drug-resistance has been reported and their action on the organism *in vitro* is stronger than that of sulphadiazine. Ampicillin is unproved in this sphere but would seem to be worthy of trial in view of its therapeutic efficacy in cases of meningitis. (Chapter 6).

Staphylococcal infections

Staphylococci are the most ubiquitous, the most adaptable but, at the same time, the most variable of all known pathogens. They accompany man and many animal species in any climate and any environment. The more crowded the community, the greater is the density and interchange of these organisms, which have as their common habitat skin and dust. They can cause almost any kind and degree of infection, from a simple boil or infected abrasion to a generalized pyaemia. If auto-infection and re-infection are minimized, many of the superficial infections caused by staphylococci are self-localizing and heal spontaneously. In these circumstances systemic therapy with antibiotics is unnecessary and, insofar as it may favour the development of drug-resistant organisms, undesirable; there is little doubt that the widespread use of penicillin G for relatively minor lesions and for prophylactic purposes in hospitals between 1945 and 1950 contributed to the spread of resistant strains by cross-infection during these years[39] and subsequently[40,41].

Many deeper abscesses in soft tissue (*e.g.* breast) can be cured by surgical drainage alone but severe or less accessible lesions (*e.g.* osteomyelitis) with *Staphylococcus aureus* are unlikely to resolve and should always receive some form of antibacterial therapy. In text-books written before the recognition of systemic penicillin as a therapeutic agent, generalized infections (septicaemia, pyaemia) are habitually described as being incurable, a description which accords well with the experience of those who had experience of major staphylococcal sepsis in pre-penicillin days. For a few lucky and, as it happened, critical years between 1944 and 1950, penicillin G reversed this prognosis.

The epidemiological impact of penicillin G upon staphylococci was therefore double-edged. The endemic and intermittently epidemic infections caused by penicillin-sensitive strains were greatly reduced in incidence and severity. On the other hand, there existed from the beginning strains of staphylococci with a relatively high natural resistance to penicillin[42,43]. The use of penicillin eliminated many sensitive strains leading, in hospitals and other communities[44,45] to an increase in penicillin-resistant strains some of which displayed high infectivity and a capacity for developing resistance to other antibiotics. The repercussions of this unfortunate story are too well known to require further description here except to say that the epidemiological clock moved backward and the hospital staphylococcus showed signs of rivalling the germs of Semmelweiss in nosocomial notoriety. Many factors were involved in this virtually selective evolution of a man-made pathogen—the ubiquity of the organism, carriers, imperfect design of hospitals and many other variables[46-49]—but it became clear that there was an all-important difference between penicillin and every other antibacterial drug in this process. Penicillin-resistance did not develop during or as a direct result of treatment of the individual case; all fully virulent and cross-infective strains of penicillin-resistant staphylococci were and are penicillinase-formers[41], the successors presumably of naturally occurring strains which either possessed the genetic information necessary for constructing the enzyme or were capable of accepting the appropriate gene by recombination or transduction[50]. The natural history of the evolutionary mechanisms which have been operating under our very eyes, aided and unaided, in this situation are still imperfectly understood but there are a few illuminating vignettes here and there:

References p. 182/184

for instance, the studies by Smith and Marples[51] which show that penicil-linase-formation may enable staphylococci to survive in the skin of hedge-hogs naturally infected by penicillin-forming dermatophytes; an experimen-tal result reported by Shilo and Citri[52] that the presence of a minority popu-lation of resistant staphylococci neutralizes by penicillinase-induction *in vivo* the action of penicillin G upon sensitive staphylococci; and the important finding by Novick[53] that penicillinase-production is controlled by a small accessory chromosome carrying other non-vital genes such as resistance to mercuric ions and erythromycin.

Since penicillinase-production was the key factor, it could have been pre-dicted—and sometimes was (Chapter 3)—that a penicillin insusceptible to the enzyme might reverse the trend. Certainly other measures to reduce cross-infection, and other antibiotics, had failed to do so[54-56]. The discovery and rapid clinical use of methicillin and the isoxazoles from 1960 onward settled the argument for the time being and demonstrated once again that a good drug, properly used, can be a powerful epidemiological tool. The organism at present is under control (see Chapters 8 and 13) and there is reason to believe that enlightened measures of ward service and hospital design[57] might serve to prevent its re-instatement. A third epidemiological phase is looming with the appearance, in several centres in Europe and a few in America*, of races of staphylococci with intrinsic, non-enzymatic resistance to the penicillinase-stable penicillins (Chapter 13). Some of these strains can cause cross-infec-tion but it is possible that they will not survive the impact of intensive therapy and strategic prophylaxis with methicillin. Meanwhile it has to be remem-bered that these new resistant strains are cross-resistant to all known deri-vatives of 6-APA and (in the writer's experience) 7-ACA so that a break-away incident might be extremely difficult to control. Their rate of increase at present is slow and even the most recently reported incidents[58] at the time of writing, are not suggestive of an epidemic problem. There is as yet no evidence that intensive prophylaxis with methicillin (unlike penicillin G) creates any problem with resistant strains of *Staph. aureus* though there is some evidence[59] that *Staph. albus* may behave differently; this organism is now increasing in importance as a cause of postoperative infection in car-diac, vascular and neurosurgical procedures.

Typical vegetatively-dividing cells of staphylococci rarely attain a level of resistance higher than 100 µg/ml of methicillin. L-forms, however, can be selectively isolated and grow in concentrations exceeding 1000 µg/ml (Ref. 60). Atypical granular colonies can also survive this concentration.

* See GRAVENKEMPER et al., J. Bact., 89 (1965) 1005.

These atypical forms of Staph. aureus are readily yielded by strains showing evidence of clinical resistance and, when isolated, appear to be unaffected by concentrations of methicillin as high as 10 mg/ml. They are also highly resistant to other forms of penicillin and to some other bactericidal antibiotics[61]. The question, therefore, arises as to whether these forms of bacteria can occur in vivo and perhaps persist in tissues or apparently-sterile lesions when typical cells can no longer be isolated. It is at present a matter of great importance to see whether or not these forms of bacteria can be isolated directly from the body or identified in infected tissue.

The infections cited above exemplify the epidemiological importance of the penicillins. For obvious reasons, preventive medicine cannot rely entirely or even mainly upon penicillins or any other drugs to attain its objectives but there is no doubt that, with some infections (staphylococcal, rheumatic, gonococcal, syphilitic) the penicillins have been more effective than any other single measure to date and often more effective than all other measures combined in preventing disease. This means that the penicillins are custodians of at least these and possibly other communicable problems and are probably irreplaceable at present in this capacity. It follows that any leakage in the penicillin barrier should be a matter of immediate epidemiological concern in the prospective sense. The mechanisms and trends underlying the resistance of gonococci and staphylococci to all forms of penicillin must be viewed in this way even if only a minority of strains are involved.

In preventive medicine, drug-dependence implies that other measures are inadequate. In the spread of pyogenic infection of open wounds, burns, respiratory tract and other situations, this is certainly true because of weaknesses in medical and nursing practice, and obsolete architecture in hospitals. Antibacterial drugs often mask these defects but, even if a drug solves some difficulties, it soon creates others, and drug-dependence should be a secondary never a primary principle in preventive procedures. With organ-transplantation, vascular prosthesis, whole-body irradiation, cytotoxic infusions and similar forms of cliff-edge therapy on the increase, it is important that chemo-prophylaxis be viewed as only one component of a systematic approach toward pathogen-free or even germ-free conditions—though the microbiological advantages of this pursuit must be weighed against the psychological disadvantages. This may also be an important consideration in dealing with the artificial atmospheres of other 20th century activities.

Finally, the epidemiological problems arising from the use of any antibacterial drugs, penicillins included, are due in part to the suppression or

References p. 182/184

even elimination of the natural flora (p. 128) especially in the respiratory and intestinal tracts. In so far as organisms in this category may be defensive, there is a need to study conditions in which the original flora can be protected or replaced. The work of Shinefield[62] and his colleagues with staphylococci, and other studies[63,64] with coliforms, suggest that this is practicable and possibly advantageous. This positive approach, though at present experimental, recalls earlier concepts that natural immunity may depend partly upon the presence of infection. In the words of an authority[65] "Nothing precise is known about the mechanism of infection immunity, even though the phenomenon has long been recognized". The same might be said about the elimination of micro-organisms in general from their natural habitat. Since we have now with the aid of drugs and other antibacterial agents entered an uncharted zone, the need for cautious microbiological soundings is more than ever necessary. At the same time, it must be remembered that any difficulties caused by the use of penicillin, even on a wide scale, are very small indeed in comparison with the benefits. If there is an epidemic, whether of venereal disease in the community or staphylococci in a hospital, chemoprophylaxis and chemotherapy, usually with one of the penicillins, are essential.

REFERENCES

1 HIRSH, H. L., ROTMAN-KAVKA, G., DOWLING, H. F. AND SWEET, L. K., *J. Amer. med. Ass.*, *133* (1947) 657.
2 FABRICANT, N. D., *Amer. J. med. Sci.*, *212* (1946) 506.
3 WEISS, J. A. AND MANHEIMS, P. J., *U.S. Nav. med. Bull.*, *46* (1946) 1711.
4 JOHNSON, ELOISE E., STOLLERMAN, G. H. AND GROSSMAN, B. J., *J. Amer. med. Ass.*, *190* (1964) 407.
5 FEINSTEIN, A. R., *New Engl. J. Med.*, *260* (1959) 697.
6 FEINSTEIN, A. R. AND SPAGNUOLO, M., *J. chron. Dis.*, *15* (1962) 623.
7 Primer on rheumatic disease, *J. Amer. med. Ass.*, *190* (1964) 425.
8 KIRBY, W. M. M., In *Antimicrobial Agents and Chemotherapy*, 1964.
9 QUOTED by OSLER, W., in *Aequanimitas*. Philadelphia, The Blakiston Comp., 1906, p. 248.
10 BOLTON, W. W., *Hygiea*, *25* (1947) 22.
11 ABERNETHY, T. J., *Trans. Stud. Coll. Phycns Philad.*, *14* (1946) 98.
12 EATON, M. D. AND VAN HERICK, W., *Amer. J. Hyg.*, *45* (1947) 82.
13 FINLAND, M., JONES, W. E., AND BARNES, MILDRED W., *J. Amer. med. Ass.*, *170* (1959) 2188.
14 *Lancet, i* (1963) 26.
15 *New Engl. J. Med.*, *268* (1963) 1141.
16 MILLER, L. F., RYTEL, M., PIERCE, W. E. AND ROSENBAUM, J. J., *J. Amer. med. Ass.*, *185* (1963) 92.
17 *Lancet, i* (1963) 346.

EPIDEMIOLOGICAL IMPACT 183

18 MEADS, M. AND FINLAND, M., *Amer. J. Syph.*, *30* (1946) 586.
19 JONES, T. R. L., DONALDSON, E. M. AND ALLEN, S. J., *Lancet, i* (1946) 526.
20 CURTIS, F. R. AND WILKINSON, P. E., *Brit. J. vener. Dis.*, *34* (1958) 70.
21 CRADOCK-WATSON, J. E., SHOOTER, R. A. AND NICOL, C. S., *Brit. med. J.*, *I* (1958) 1091.
22 Medical Research Council, *Interim report of Committee on penicillin-resistant gono-cocci*, 1961.
23 KING, A., Recent Advances in Venereology. Churchill, London, 1964.
24 MOORE, M. B., SHORT, D. H., MATHESON, T. F., KNOX, J. M. AND VANDERSTOEP, E. M., *Publ. Hlth Rep. (Wash.)*, *78* (1963) 261.
25 SOCHUS, R. H., LUCERO, F. M. AND MEKALOJIZH, R. J., *J. Amer. med. Ass.*, *177* (1961) 121.
26 STRATFORD, B. C., *Med. J. Australia*, *49* (1963) 414.
27 WILLCOX, R. R., In BRUMFITT, W. AND WILLIAMS, J. D. (Eds), *Proceedings of Conference on Therapy with the New Penicillins, Postgrad. med. J.*, *Suppl.*, *40* (1964) 202.
28 NICOL, C. S., *Brit. J. vener. Dis.*, *40* (1964) 96.
29 KING, A. J., *Prescribers Journal*, *4* (1964) 35.
30 D'ALLESSANDRO, G. AND DARDONONI, L., *Amer. J. Syph.*, *37* (1953) 137.
31 KING, A. J., *Lancet, i* (1958) 651.
32 *Amer. J. Publ. Hlth*, *53* (1963) 1835.
33 *Syphilis: modern diagnosis and management.* Report by U.S. Public Health Service. Dept. of Health, Education, and Welfare, Washington, 1960.
34 WILLCOX, R. R., *Curr. Med. Drugs*, *4* (1964) 3.
35 World Health Organization, Expert Committee on Venereal disease and treponematoses. 4th and 5th reports, Nos. 63 and 190. World Health Organization, Geneva, 1953; 1960.
36 GUTHE, T., *Bull. Wld Hlth Org.*, *19* (1958) 405.
37 MILLER, J. W., SIESS, E. E., FELDMAN. H, A., SILVERMAN, C. AND FRANK, P., *J. Amer. med. Ass.*, *186* (1963) 139.
38 IVLER, D., LEEDOM, J. M., THRUPP, L. D., WEHRLE, P. F., PORTNOY, B. AND MATHIES, A. W., to be published, (1964).
39 BARBER, MARY, *J. Path. Bact.*, *59* (1947) 373.
40 WALLMARK, G. AND FINLAND, M., *J. Amer. med. Ass.*, *175* (1961) 886.
41 *Lancet, i* (1961) 886.
42 KIRBY, W. M. M., *Science*, *99* (1944) 452.
43 KIRBY, W. M. M., *J. clin. Invest.*, *24* (1945) 165.
44 ROODYN, L., *Proc. roy. Soc. Med.*, *49* (1955) 263.
45 WALLMARK, G. AND FINLAND, M., *J. Amer. med. Ass.*, *175* (1961) 150.
46 BLOWERS, R., MASON, G. A., WALLACE, K. R., AND WALTON, M., *Lancet, ii* (1955) 786.
47 SPINK, W. W., *Ann. N.Y. Acad. Sci.*, *65* (1956) 175.
48 SHOOTER, R. A., SMITH, M. A., GRIFFITHS, J. D., BROWN, M. E. A., WILLIAMS, R. E. O., RIPPON, J. E. AND JEVONS, M. P., *Brit. med. J.*, *I* (1958) 607.
49 HASSAL, J. E. AND ROUNTREE, P. M., *Lancet, i* (1959) 213.
50 RITZ, H. L. AND BALDWIN, J. N., *Proc. Soc. exp. Biol. (N.Y.)*, *107* (1961) 678.
51 SMITH, J. M. P. AND MARPLES, MARY J., *Nature*, *201* (1964) 844.
52 SHILO, M. AND CITRI, N., *Brit. J. exp. Path.*, *45* (1964) 192.
53 NOVICK, R., *J. gen. Microbiol.*, *33* (1963) 121.
54 *Lancet, ii* (1955) 755.
55 GILLESPIE, W. A., *Med. J. S. W.*, *73* (1958) 56.
56 ROUNTREE, P. M., HARRINGTON, M., LOEWENTHAL, J. AND GYE, R., *Lancet, ii* (1960) 1.
57 BULLOCK, W. E., HALL, J. W., SPINK, W. W., DAMSKY, L. J., GREEN, V. W., VESLEY, D. AND BAUER, H., *Ann. intern. Med.*, *60* (1964) 777.
58 STILLE, W. AND HIRSCH, H. A., *Münch. med. Wschr.*, *106* (1964) 1528.

[59] STEWART, G. T., *Brit. med. J., I* (1961) 863.
[60] KAGAN, B. M., MARTIN, E. R. AND STEWART, G. T., *Nature, 203* (1964) 1031.
[61] KAGAN, B. M., "Staphylococci: ecologic perspectives." *Ann. N.Y. Acad. Sci.,* (1964) to be published.
[62] SHINEFIELD, H. R., RIBBLE, J. C., EICHENWALD, H. F., BORIS, H. M. AND SUTHERLAND, J. M., *Amer. J. Dis. Child., 105* (1963) 683.
[63] SEARS, H. J., JANES, H., SALOUM, R., BROWNLEE, I. AND LAMOUREAUX, L. F., *J. Bact., 71* (1956) 370.
[64] STEWART, G. T., HOLT, R. J., COLES, H. M. T. AND BHAT, K. M., *J. Hyg. (Lond.), 62* (1964) 39.
[65] DUBOS, R., *Amer. J. Dis. Child., 105* (1963) 643.

Chapter 16

CEPHALOSPORINS

It has been known since 1945 that moulds of the species *Cephalosporium* produce antibiotics possessing some activity against gram-positive and gram-negative bacteria. Like penicillin, these antibiotics were described and examined unobtrusively, first in Sardinia by Brotzu[1] who made the discovery, and then at Oxford by Florey and his colleagues[2]. Several antibiotics with differing properties were isolated from *Cephalosporium* spp. These were named at first cephalosporins C, N and P. Independently, American workers[3] in 1951 isolated an antibiotic which they named synnematin B from *Cephalosporium salmosynnematum*. This antibiotic was found to be identical with cephalosporin N and is in fact a penicillin (penicillin N) with a straight D-(4-amino-4-carboxybutyl) side chain[4]. It is active against some gram-negative bacteria (p. 101) but has never been tested pharmacologically or as a therapeutic agent sufficiently thoroughly to establish its position. Cephalosporin P is now known to be a group of tetracyclic compounds of steroid structure[5] with some activity against gram-positive micrococci.

Cephalosporin C resembled penicillin in possessing a fused β-lactam ring but contained two oxygen and two carbon atoms more, and had D-α-amino-adipic acid in the side-chain. The full structure was elucidated at Oxford by ingenious chemical[6] and crystallographic[7] analyses which defined the positions of all the atoms in the molecule thereby adding an important increment to knowledge of structure-activity relationship.

$$\underset{\bar{O}_2C}{\overset{H_3\overset{+}{N}\diagdown D}{}}\!\!\!\!CH.CH_2.CH_2.CH_2.CO.NH.\underset{7}{CH}\text{——}\underset{6}{CH}\overset{S}{\diagdown}{}_2CH_2$$

The nucleus of cephalosporin C consists of a 6-membered dihydrothiazine ring, in place of the 5-membered thiazolidine ring of the penicillins, fused to a β-lactam ring. This nucleus (7-amino-cephalosporanic acid, 7-ACA) contains structures (shown in heavy type in the formula) which are present also in 6-amino-penicillanic acid (6-APA)including a peptide linkage (CO:NH) vulnerable to hydrolysis by amidase[8] and a carbonyl (C = O) group whose stretching vibration causes strong absorption of infra-red light at 5.61 μ (1760 cm^{-1}). Loss of this absorption band indicates opening of the β-lactam ring; this can be used to detect specific hydrolysis of cephalosporin as well as of penicillin derivatives by β-lactamase[9]. The cephalosporins are in general less susceptible than penicillin G or ampicillin to hydrolysis by β-lactamase from staphylococci or B. cereus but are readily hydrolysed by enzymes from certain gram-negative bacilli, one of which, from Aerobacter cloacae, has been reported[10] as having selective affinity for the cephalosporin molecule and has been designated "Cephalosporinase". The amino-adipic acid side chain of penicillin N lessens susceptibility to β-lactamase from staphylococci or B. cereus by about half but cephalosporin C is very much less susceptible to hydrolysis (V max approximately 10^{-3}–10^{-4} times that for penicillin G). The phenylacetyl derivative of 7-ACA retains this resistance and is, like cephalosporin C, an effective inhibitor of the action of the enzyme from B. cereus on penicillin G. Competitive inhibition of hydrolysis with the phenylacetyl and other derivatives of 7-ACA as inhibitor, and penicillin N as substrate, is of the same degree as that occurring with cephalosporin C as inhibitor and penicillin G as substrate. Hence it would appear[11] that the affinity of different N-acyl derivatives of 7-ACA for β-lactamase from B. cereus is similar to that of corresponding derivatives of 6-APA. But, with staphylococcal β-lactamase, cephalosporin C does not inhibit hydrolysis of penicillin G appreciably though its phenylacetyl derivative does, more so with penicillin G than with penicillin N as substrate. The affinities of N-acyl derivatives of 6-APA and 7-ACA for staphylococcal β-lactamase are therefore greatly increased if the charged amino-adipolyl side-chain is replaced by a benzyl group.

The anti-staphylococcal activity of cephalosporin C is relatively low but it has some action against streptococci and certain gram-negative bacilli, and is remarkably non-toxic in experimental animals. Despite the similarity in structure and in other biological properties, cephalosporin C and its benzyl derivatives are not cross allergenic with 6-APA and its main derivatives in subjects who are hypersensitive to penicillins[12]. This distinction presumably depends upon the presence of a thiazolidine ring or conjugate as an antigenic determinant in the penicilloyl hapten.

These properties, together with the prospect of modifying the biological activity of the 7-ACA molecule by a greater range of substituents, evoked widespread interest in the cephalosporins. But, for some years, this interest remained academic since none of the derivatives prepared showed a sufficiently high order of therapeutic activity to warrant clinical trial. The advent of the new penicillins from 1959 onward diverted interest to 6-APA. The Oxford research team however continued their fundamental research upon 7-ACA and it is to them and to a few manufacturers (chiefly Glaxo and Eli Lilly) that the advancement of this subject is due. Early attempts to modify the molecule were discouraging, for the N-acyl derivatives of 7-ACA were usually 5–10 times weaker in antibacterial activity than the corresponding derivatives of 6-APA[11]. But 7-ACA can be substituted in the acetoxy-methyl group attached to the dihydrothiazine ring, as well as in the 7-position, so it has potentially a wider prospect for biosynthetic modification if its other useful properties can be retained. The first useful step in this direction came when Abraham[11] and his colleagues reacted cephalosporin C with pyridine to form the first of a new series of C_A compounds with higher antibacterial activity, especially against staphylococci. These compounds are substituted in the dihydrothiazine ring but some heightening of antibacterial activity also occurs, as stated above, with replacement of the natural α-aminoadipolyl side chain in the 7-position. The first derivative of therapeutic importance was in fact the sodium salt of 7-(thiophene-2-acetamido)-cephalosporanic acid (Cephalothin) which is active in vitro against many gram-positive and gram-negative pathogens[13,14]. This drug is now marketed by Eli Lilly. It is not well absorbed when given orally but is well-tolerated when given parenterally and freely distributed in the tissues[15], including the placenta, amniotic fluid, foetal blood, aqueous humour, milk and CSF of experimental animals. Elimination by the renal tubules is rapid, and can be blocked by probenecid.

Clinical work on Cephalothin

Studies in man show that doses of 0.5–1.0 g can be given safely to adults every 6 h by the intramuscular route for several weeks[16,17]. This dosage produces serum concentrations which are bactericidal to many organisms, without cumulative effect. Doses of 1 g cause pain at the site of injection; otherwise, the only suggestions of toxicity so far reported are eosinophilia (in about 14% of children, according to one report[18], occasional maculopopular rashes, urticaria and elevation of serum transaminase[19]. In children (ref. 18) the dosage is 10–14 mg/kg/day and there is evidence[20] that this, or higher dosage can be given with impunity to newborn and premature babies.

References p. 191/192

When given to mothers immediately before delivery, the drug can be detected in cord blood at levels of a quarter to half the concentration in maternal blood.

Used in this way, and subject to sensitivity tests on all organisms isolated, there is now ample evidence[16-23] that cephalothin is effective when given intramuscularly or intravenously in the treatment of infections, in various sites, due to penicillin-resistant staphylococci, streptococci (groups A, C and D), pneumococci, *E. coli*, *Proteus* spp., the *Aerobacter-klebsiella* group and possibly other rods such as paracolon spp., and *Clostridium perfringens*. When the organism is relatively insensitive—as in the case of many of the gram-negative rods—or when infection is severe, large doses seem to be well-tolerated: Weinstein[23] and his colleagues found that 4 g per day cured a patient with a generalised staphylococcal infection which had not responded to 2 g per day, and they quote another patient who received 24 g daily for two weeks without apparent toxicity. Other workers[22] found a daily dosage of 6 g effective in septicaemia due to *B. alcaligenes faecalis* but 12 g ineffective in septicaemia caused by *Aerobacter aerogenes*, though the organism was killed by 2 μg/ml *in vitro*. The drug is inactive against *Ps. pyocyanea* and unproved against *Salmonella* spp., some of which are sensitive *in vitro*. Clinical failures are reported mainly in patients with severe or complicated infections but Heitler *et al*[18] report failures in three uncomplicated respiratory and one urinary infection; they also note that pneumococci persist in naso-pharyngeal swabs during treatment, despite their high sensitivity to the drug. Drug-resistance does not seem to have been encountered but in a number of cases the infecting organisms have persisted during or after treatment, and there is as yet no detailed data about these. Gram-negative rods vary widely in sensitivity and the bactericidal effect of the drug, even upon those classed as sensitive at 5–10 μg/ml, is often incomplete, so it will be surprising if resistant mutants are lacking.

Cephaloridine

This derivative of 7-ACA is

7-[(2-thienyl) acetamido]-3-(1-pyridylmethyl)-3 cephem-4-carboxylic acid betaine.

It thus combines the thienylacetamido-substituent of cephalothin with a pyridine ring in the 3-position, which was found by Abraham and his colleagues (see above) to increase anti-bacterial activity and also to stabilise this part of the molecule in mammalian tissues[24]. The drug is very soluble in water, slightly acid but stable at pH 4.5–5.0 for weeks in the dark at 4° C. The antibacterial spectrum is similar to that of cephalothin though intrinsic bactericidal activity is slightly but regularly higher against most organisms, gram-positive and gram-negative[25]. In pharmacological behaviour and lack of toxicity in animals it is also very similar to cephalothin[26]. Renal excretion is rapid, accounting for 50–80% of an injected dose, but the fate of the unexcreted moiety is uncertain; a small residue can be detected in the livers of treated rats[27] but there is no other cumulative trend and no active metabolites can be detected in the urine or tissues. In tissue cultures of human fibroblasts and other cells, concentrations of 100 μg/ml cause some retardation of growth but cytotoxic effects are not seen until the concentration rises to 500–1000 μg/ml and, even at these high concentrations, there is no interference with the respiration of hepatic cells[27] nor is a metabolite detectable when tissues are treated with these concentrations. This may be due to the stabilising effect of the 3-substituent, for cephalothin is attacked in tissues by an esterase which hydrolyses it to an o-desacetyl metabolite, detectible in serum and urine[15].

Clinical studies in man [27,28] confirm that cephaloridine in doses of 500 mg 6-hourly in adults or 10–30 mg/kg/day in children produces bactericidal levels in the serum and is well-tolerated when given by intramuscular, or intravenous injections. Intrathecal (50 mg) and intraventricular (2 mg) injections are also acceptable. Serum levels after intramuscular injection are very variable—2–30 μg/ml after 15 min, 1–70 μg/ml after1 h, 0–10 μg/ml after 4–6 h.

At the time of writing, the only two published reports[27,28] refer to a total of 68 patients with infections due to the pyogenic cocci or to *E. coli, Aerobacter aerogenes, Proteus* spp. and *Clostridium perfringens* (1 case). All of these infections were however severe; many had resisted therapy with other drugs and several had septicaemia or mixed infection. The overall results indicate a good, sometimes impressive, clinical result in at least two-thirds of the cases treated, failures being associated only with complications and anatomical deformities, especially in the renal tract. The effect against pyogenic coccal infections is comparable to that of the penicillins but the most impressive property of the drug is undoubtedly its capacity to eliminate or control severe urinary and systemic infections with certain gram-negative bacilli, especially *Aerobacter aerogenes* which is notoriously difficult to treat except with toxic drugs like Kanamycin. Like the other cephalosporins, cephaloridine is not cross-allergenic with the penicillins in sensitised subjects.

Place of the cephalosporins in therapy

Enough information is now available to assign to cephalothin and cephaloridine a proved place as broad-spectrum agents with higher intrinsic activity than the tetracyclines or chloramphenicol against all susceptible species and higher activity than ampicillin against the *Klebsiella-aerogenes* group. In infections due to this group of organisms, the two cephalosporins might now fairly be regarded as drugs of first choice, provided adequate sensitivity tests are performed, for there is wide variation within species. The cephalosporins are also relatively insusceptible to β-lactamase, cephaloridine being more stable than cephalothin to this enzyme from most staphylococci, though slightly less stable to both the β-lactamase and amidase from some coliforms[27]. On all other grounds, cephaloridine would appear to be more active and more stable metabolically than cephalothin but, at the time of writing, cephalothin has had extensive clinical trials with consistent results, whereas cephaloridine is still undergoing preliminary evaluation. Both drugs have the disadvantage of being unsuitable for oral medication and it is to be hoped that further biosynthetic modification will be attempted, perhaps at the α-carbon atom, to overcome this fault. As things stand, these two derivatives are by far the best of a number which have been prepared. They fill a gap in the therapy of some gram-negative infections and are indicated for immediate use in patients known or thought to be allergic to the penicillins. It is possible that the cephalosporins will induce their own specific hypersensitivities but this is unproved as yet nor is there any indication of whether or not a similar degradation with antigenic conjugation occurs.

The mode of action of the cephalosporins upon staphylococci appears to be biochemically close, possibly identical with that of penicillin[29]. The strong bactericidal action on gram-negative bacilli is unexplained; the morphological changes are less pronounced than those produced by penicillin G or ampicillin, even when the organisms are more susceptible *in vitro*[27]. This activity will be extremely difficult to probe without close attention to metabolic variations within any given bacterial species in view of the inconsistency of action against any one species and the susceptibility of the drugs to inactivating enzymes. This variability is of importance also in practical therapy, for superinfection with resistant organisms can occur readily, especially in the treatment of chronic infections of the urinary tract. These resistant organisms may in some instances be of the same species and are then difficult to differentiate from drug-resistant mutants of the original species which may also emerge during therapy with cephaloridine. *Ps. pyocyanea* is inherently resistant to all forms of cephalosporin and can also cause super-infection[23,27]. Methicillin-resistant staphylococci are also sometimes resistant to all available forms of cephalosporin.

The value of the cephalosporins is therefore reasonably definite as far as their use in refractory gram-negative infections are concerned, and in the treatment of patients with hypersensitivity to penicillin. They are perhaps the immediate successors to penicillin in speed of action and non-toxicity, but they cannot as yet be used speculatively. Their main potential lies in the possibility of greater modification of the 7-ACA than of the 6-APA nucleus, a potential which is immensely heightened by the advance in understanding of structure-activity brought about by their discovery and molecular analysis. From now on, the penicillins and cephalosporins have to be regarded in the scientific sense at least as belonging to a widening range of antibiotics of fused dipeptide structure with a common β-lactam ring and closely-related biological properties. Collectively, these β-lactam antibiotics show signs of controlling a far greater range of bacteria than any other group of identifiable substances. It is impossible now to consider the action or modification of penicillins without close attention to the behaviour of the cephalosporins and *vice-versa*. This is the last chapter in this book but it could equally serve as an opening to a new story in chemotherapy, in which systematic chemical knowledge of structure and mode of action precede proof of therapeutic action. It will be interesting to see if this makes a difference for, if it does, prediction will at last have ousted empiricism in one branch of applied biology.

REFERENCES

[1] BROTZU, G., *Lav. Ist. Ig. Cagliari*, (1948).
[2] BURTON, H. S. AND ABRAHAM, E. P., *Biochem. J.*, *50* (1951) 168.
[3] GOTTSHAL, R. Y., ROBERTS, J. M., PORTWOOD, L. M. AND JENNINGS, J. C., *Proc. Soc. exp. Biol. (N.Y.)*, *76* (1951) 307.
[4] NEWTON, G. G. F. AND ABRAHAM, E. P., *Biochem. J.*, *58* (1954) 94.
[5] BURTON, H. S., ABRAHAM, E. P. AND CARDWELL, H. M. E., *Biochem. J.*, *62* (1956) 171.
[6] ABRAHAM, E. P. AND NEWTON, G. G. F., *Biochem. J.*, *79* (1961) 337.
[7] HODGKIN, D. AND MASLEN, E. N., *Biochem. J.*, *79* (1961) 393.
[8] HOLT, R. J. AND STEWART, G. T., *J. gem. Microbiol.*, *36* (1964) 203.
[9] HOLT, R. J. AND STEWART, G. T., *Biochim. Biophys. Acta*, *100* (1964) 235.
[10] FLEMING, P. C., GOLDNER, H. AND GLASS, D. G., *Lancet*, *i* (1963) 1399.

[11] ABRAHAM, E. P., *Pharmacol. Rev.*, *14* (1962) 473.
[12] STEWART, G. T., *Lancet*, *i* (1961) 509.
[13] BONIECE, W. S., WICK, W. E., HOLMES, D. M. AND REDMAN, C., *J. Bact.*, *84* (1962) 1292.
[14] GODZESKI, C. W., BRIER, G. AND PAVEY, D. E., *Appl. Microbiol.*, *11* (1963) 122.
[15] CHENG-CHUN, LEE AND ANDERSON, R. C., *Antimicrobial Agents and Chemotherapy*, (1962) 695.
[16] ANDERSON, K. N. AND PETERSDORF, R. G., *Antimicrobial Agents and Chemotherapy*, (1962) 724.
[17] HERELL, W. E., BALOWS, A. AND BECKER, JEAN, *Clin. Pharmacol. Ther.*, *4* (1963) 709.
[18] HEITLER, M. S., ISENBERG, H. D., KARELITS, S., ACS, HEDDA AND MILLER, MAXINE, *Antimicrobial Agents and Chemotherapy*, (1962) 261.
[19] RILEY, H. D., BRACKEN, E. C. AND FLUX, M., *Antimicrobial Agents and Chemotherapy*, (1963) 716.
[20] REICHELDERFER, L. C. AND REICHELDERFER, J. E., *Clin. Med.*, *71* (1964) 2.
[21] PHILSON, J. R., CLANCY, C. F. AND ALEXANDER, J. D., *Antimicrobial Agents and Chemotherapy*, (1962) 267.
[22] WALTERS, E. W., ROMANSKY, M. J. AND JOHNSON, A. C., *Antimicrobial Agents and Chemotherapy*, (1964) 247.
[23] WEINSTEIN, L., KAPLAN, K. AND TE-WEN, CHANG, *J. Amer. med. Ass.*, *189* (1964) 829.
[24] O'CALLAGHAN, CYNTHIA H. AND MUGGLETON, P. W., *Biochem. J.*, *89* (1963) 304.
[25] MUGGLETON, P. W., O'CALLAGHAN, CYNTHIA H. AND STEVENS, W. K., *Brit. med. J.*, *II* (1961) 1234.
[26] CURRIE, J. P. AND TOMICH, E. G., to be published, 1964.
[27] STEWART, G. T. AND HOLT, R. J., *Lancet*, *ii* (1964) 1305.
[28] MURDOCH, J. McC., SPEIRS, C. F., GEDDES, A. M. AND WALLACE, R. T., *Brit. med. J.*, *II* (1964) 1238.
[29] TE-WEN, CHANG AND WEINSTEIN, L., *Science*, *143* (1964) 807.

AUTHOR INDEX

Zaremba, E. A., 59
Zilliken, F., 89, 93
Zinder, N. D., 141

Zinneman, H. H., 68
Zolla, Susan, 92
Zylka, W. von, 56–58, 62

SUBJECT INDEX